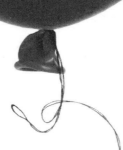

Working on
Health
Communication
Nova Corcoran

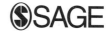

⑤SAGE

Los Angeles | London | New Delhi
Singapore | Washington DC

SAGE Publications Ltd
1 Oliver's Yard
55 City Road
London EC1Y 1SP

SAGE Publications Inc.
2455 Teller Road
Thousand Oaks, California 91320

SAGE Publications India Pvt Ltd
B 1/11 Mohan Cooperative Industrial Area
Mathura Road, New Delhi 110 044
India

SAGE Publications Asia-Pacific Pte Ltd
33 Pekin Street#02-01
Far East Square
Singapore 048763

Library of Congress Control Number: 2010922796

British Library Cataloguing in Publication data

A catalogue record for this book is available from the British Library

ISBN 978-1-84787-922-6
ISBN 978-1-84787-923-3 (pbk)

Typeset by C&M Digitals (P) Ltd., Chennai, India
Printed by MPG Books Group, Bodmin, Cornwall
Printed on paper from sustainable resources

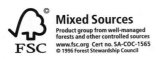

Mixed Sources
Product group from well-managed
forests and other controlled sources
www.fsc.org Cert no. SA-COC-1565
© 1996 Forest Stewardship Council

Contents

List of figures

List of tables

Author's acknowledgements

Thank you to all the students at the University of East London, especially those in the Communication and Health class for their enthusiasm and ideas.

I would like to acknowledge my contacts at Sage for orientating me in the right directions. I would like to thank friends and family who supplied me with ideas, sanity, time out, child-minding, food and proof reading. A special mention goes to Ben Scott, Calvin Moorley, Joanne Middleton, Emma Halliday and my parents. A big thank you to Ostyn and Huxley for keeping me grounded in the real world and being such good sleepers. A final thank you goes to the Dockland Light Railway service as all the time spent on their trains gave me my best ideas!

Publisher's acknowledgements

Every effort has been made to trace all the copyright holders, but if any have been accidentally overlooked the publishers will be happy to make the necessary changes at the first opportunity.

Department for Transport for Figure 5.1: Drug driving: your eyes will give you away glasses (DfT 2009).

Department for Transport for Figure 6.1: 'Live with it' (DfT 2009) road safety campaign poster.

Department of Health for Figure 6.2: Change4Life (DH 2009) poster.

QUIT for Figure 6.5: QUIT (2007) 'Don't over do it' poster.

Introduction

Campaigns are central to the development of public health interventions. There is a growing dependence on campaigns as a primary strategy for public health interventions (Kreps and Maibach 2009). All health promotion and public health interventions include some form of communication (McKenzie et al. 2005) and good communication is essential in the design of campaigns to promote health or prevent ill health.

The notion of communication is changing and campaign designers are now faced with a wealth of new media channels to use in their work. The popularity of electronic media, such as social networking channels and internet-based television, is encouraging practitioners to think creatively about campaign design.

Even campaigns in the political sphere are changing the way people think about issues that impact on the communities in which they live. Abroms and Lefebure (2009) note that in President Obama's successful presidential election campaign, use was made of a campaign website, a campaign TV channel (YouTube), social network sites, mobile phones, and unofficial campaign materials (such as blogs and students' websites). The exposure levels achieved by the campaign were vast. For example, by November 2008 1,700 videos of Obama had been uploaded to YouTube and viewed over 18 million times. Abroms and Lefebure suggest Obama's political campaigns provide four possible lessons for health campaigns. They are:

- consider new media such as social network sites, blogs, or Short Messaging Services (SMS) on mobile phones;
- encourage 'horizontal' communication, such as peer-to-peer and user-generated messages;
- use new media for small acts of engagement (such as sending e-mails) that help to build relationships;
- use social media to facilitate, rather than replace, interpersonal grassroots work.

These lessons suggest that traditional health campaigns need to be reconceived in light of the availability of new media and people's communication preferences.

'Communication' refers to the exchange of information, thoughts, or feelings between individuals or groups (The Communications Network 2008). Such exchanges take place through channels of communication. These channels may be grouped into four categories, namely, (1) intrapersonal; (2) interpersonal; (3) organizational; and (4) community. These are hierarchical in nature, with

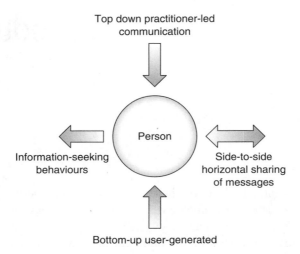

Top down practitioner-led
communication

Person

Information-seeking
behaviours

Side-to-side
horizontal sharing
of messages

Bottom-up user-generated

Figure 0.1   A new model of communication
Source: Adapted from Thackery and Neiger (2009).

interpersonal (one-to-one communication) reaching the smallest number of people and community reaching the whole population.

Current research suggests that combining both interpersonal or intrapersonal communication with communication at organizational or community level is more effective than using mass media alone – a point that we discuss further in Chapter 5.

The changing nature of communication implies that older (sequential) communication models consisting of: (1) a sender; (2) a message; and (3) a receiver are no longer appropriate. This is in part because they do not include a mechanism for feedback (or responding to that feedback) and partly because of the changing nature of communication. Today, the health communication process is multi-directional as the general population actively seeks information from the immediate, accessible formats. Thackery and Neiger (2009) have therefore proposed a new model of communication, as shown in Figure 0.1.

This model assumes that communication may be expert-generated, i.e. from top down (as in traditional models of communication), or user-generated, i.e bottom up, or side-to-side (i.e. horizontal). The population actively seeks information and this becomes part of this communication cycle. Although Thackery and Neiger suggest the application of this model in social marketing, this model is also appropriate for health campaigns.

Other authors emphasize the importance of horizontal sharing of information (Abroms and Lefebure 2009). Traditional media is often considered a one-way source (Gray et al. 2005) but health communication campaigns should no longer rely on such models. They need to consider their target audiences and the context in which they live their lives. The continual nature of communication is often ignored by campaigns: the Department of Health notes that campaigns are often 'inconsistent, uncoordinated and out of step' (DH 2004: 21) with the lived experience of their target audiences.

There are a number of reasons why campaigns may fail to be effective. Atkin notes that in some campaigns audience members are lost because messages can be 'offensive, disturbing, boring, stale, preachy, confusing, irritating, misleading, irrelevant, uninformative, useless, unbelievable or unmotivating' (2001: 51). This is also true for the whole campaign process. If planning models are confusing, target groups irrelevant, materials useless, or evaluations misleading, then communication campaigns are doomed to failure. The design, implementation, and evaluation of a communication campaign can be challenging and practitioners may need to develop a number of new skills to ensure that they can design and execute effective, suitable, appropriate campaigns.

A number of important factors are involved in the design of behaviour change campaigns at population, community and individual level (NICE 2007). These include planning interventions carefully, taking into account the wider contexts of communities, and evaluating work. In addition, needs assessments, acknowledging social and cultural contexts, specifying theory and models for delivery, considering barriers to change, noting time scales and setting out evaluation plans are all essential in the planning of any campaign. We also need to consider material design, message formulation and methods of delivery. There are some similarities in the NICE (2007) guidelines to recommendations first noted by Myhre and Flora (2000) and reiterated by Noar et al. (2009). The authors note that formative research, segmentation of audiences, targeted message design, effective channels for communication, high message exposure and evaluation are principles that should be followed in campaigns.

THIS BOOK

This textbook provides a practical guide to communication campaigns and their design, implementation, and evaluation. It covers areas recommended by NICE (2007) and Noar et al. (2009) alongside other key areas in health campaigns. If communication campaigns can be planned, implemented and evaluated carefully, the likelihood of an effective campaign is much higher. To help you achieve this aim, this book examines which steps need to be taken in the design of communication campaigns and the best way to undertake these.

This book has a strong academic focus. Its approach aims to help practitioners gain *practical* theoretical knowledge, by using a mixture of activities and case studies. In addition, the final chapter includes case studies of health campaigns to give examples of current good practice in communication.

The book is divided into eight chapters. The chapters aim to take into account the range of areas that practitioners will encounter when designing, implementing and evaluating communication campaigns. Each chapter includes a number of activities and case studies. The activity discussions are found at the back of this textbook and are designed to give the reader examples of model answers for these activities. There is also a glossary at the end of the book. All terms in the glossary have been highlighted in italic in the text on their first appearance, and the symbol >> appears in the margin.

Outline of content

Chapter 1 identifies the role of planning models in the design of campaigns. It considers a range of models that can be used to plan campaigns in practice. This chapter includes both basic and complex planning models, as well as examples of these planning models in practice.

Chapter 2 considers the foundations of campaigns. This includes formulating aims and objectives, identifying stakeholders and establishing the role of theoretical models in planning campaigns. A selection of theoretical models are discussed to illustrate the importance of theory in campaign design.

Chapter 3 examines the factors involved in the campaign design process, such as researching health issues and identifying settings and locations for campaigns. It also discusses the writing of campaign rationales and the collection of data to inform campaign planning.

Chapter 4 analyses the target groups in the campaign context. Target groups' social and psychological characteristics such as age, sex, ethnicity, culture and religion are considered alongside questions concerning knowledge, attitudes, beliefs and values. Ways to tailor information to different target groups are also considered.

Chapter 5 examines communication channels in campaigns. This includes the role of interpersonal, intrapersonal, organizational and community channels of communication. Ways to utilize mass media and electronic media are also discussed.

Chapter 6 outlines the steps to be taken when designing a print-based resource. This chapter works through eight steps in the design process and considers the role of readability, typography, interactive features and visuals. This chapter also considers the design of messages and message framing.

Chapter 7 considers the role of evaluation. It highlights the evaluation cycle of process, impact and outcomes evaluation. It considers formative evaluation and cost evaluation. Consideration is also given to evaluation techniques that are specifically linked to media such as monitoring activities and media analysis as well as unconventional ways of evaluating.

Chapter 8 provides a summary of the main themes and recommendations of this textbook. It also provides an outline of ten campaigns in order to assist practitioners in the design, implementation and evaluation of their own campaigns.

This book draws on journals and communication information sources from around the world. The areas it draws on are being constantly updated (for example, information technology and new media), where reliance on current information is essential. It is hoped that, by using sources from journals and existing health-related organizations, this textbook will provide practitioners with an up-to-date compendium of ideas and practices to assist in the design, implementation and evaluation of health-related communication campaigns.

Planning campaigns

Planning is essential to ensure success in health campaigns. This chapter will highlight the role of planning in the design of health campaigns and consider why planning is integral to success. This chapter will identify four planning models: (1) the nine-step model; (2) the Total Process Planning Model; (3) PRECEDE-PROCEED; and (4) Intervention Mapping. These are taken from various disciplines connected to health and can be applied to health campaigns. This chapter will evaluate these models and consider how they can work in a practical context.

This chapter aims to:

- explore the rationale for using planning models in campaign planning and design
- identify a selection of planning models that can be used in the design of campaigns
- apply theoretical aspects of planning models to health communication practice

PLANNING

Planning can contribute to a health campaign by helping to:

- identify the main problem and solution;
- identify the correct approach;
- ensure effective resource use and allocation;
- avoid unwanted outcomes.

Practitioners need to ensure that, in any campaign, both the main problem and its solution are identified. Russell et al. (2003) suggest that if the problem is not described accurately, then factors including the inability to identify an alternative solution may not be possible. Tones and Green (2004: 109) suggest that 'the overall purpose of systematic planning is to identify goals and the most effective means of achieving them'. Planning therefore can ensure success. Godin et al. (2007), in their review of the planning process in STI and HIV campaigns, emphasize that planned campaigns are more likely to be successful. Planning not only helps to organize theories and ideas, but also ensures correct identification of a problem and a solution.

Approaches vary between campaigns. Planning assists the selection of the most appropriate approach. For example, an accident prevention campaign aimed at young children will use a different approach to a campaign that aims to increase knowledge in adults of an infectious disease. There is no single general campaign that can be applied to all health issues or all target groups. There can be considerable differences between campaigns, especially in relation to applicability and transferability of theory into practice (Wang et al. 2005; Corcoran 2007b; see also Chapter 2). Evidence from research in one campaign may not translate well into practice in another campaign.

Planning also helps to ensure that resources are used effectively. Douglas et al. (2007) indicate that failure to demonstrate a planned approach can mean there is a risk that your topic will not be given priority, and thus funding or resources may be allocated elsewhere. They also note that systematic planning can ensure resources are used effectively. From the budget-holders' or stakeholders' perspectives, planning ensures value for money and minimizes misdirected time, spending and resources. Planning is essential in ensuring any problems identified are addressed in the preliminary phases to try and eliminate factors such as misdirected messages, or administration failures.

One of the problems of campaigns is the risk of unexpected or unintended consequences, for example, a campaign may run out of resources. Moreover, there is some evidence to suggest that campaigns may have a boomerang effect (for an example, see the section on fear appeals in Chapter 6). In addition, some authors suggest campaigns can have unintentional, negative, impacts. Lee (2007) indicates that some sexual *health promotion* misses its audience with men who have sex with men, possibly in part due to the advertising imagery used having unintended consequences. Effective planning may help to reduce this risk, especially through the application of planning models.

Activity 1.1:   Unplanned outcomes

You have been working on a campaign to reduce high dietary fat intake in a group of overweight young teenagers. The main messages link appearance and feeling good with eating less fat.

1 What possible positive effects could this campaign have and what possible negative effects could this campaign have on the target group?

PLANNING MODELS

Planning need not be static, rigid or fixed. It does, however, need to be systematic (Douglas et al. 2007). Health *communication* is generally based on systematic planning models drawn from health promotion and *public health* practice. It can be argued that working to a planning model may restrict creativity and imagination in the campaign process, but on the contrary, planning models help ensure that the imaginative and creative process is developed as appropriately as possible. Horst et al. (2009) indicate the importance of adapting campaign planning to prevailing conditions. For example, their project changed elements of the original project in response to new information regarding drug toxicity, decreases of workload, and the changing realities of HIV care. A practitioner therefore needs to view planning as an adaptable process that is flexible enough to change to meet the changing realities of day-to-day health practice.

Effective planning may be based on a variety of models. 'Models are the means by which structure and organization are given to the planning process' (McKenzie et al. 2005: 15). This is not to say that a planning model is rigid and inflexible, but is more a framework that ensures everything you want to happen actually does happen. Although campaigns can take place without a planning model to guide them, the risk of the campaign not meeting outcomes, going over budget or not anticipating avoidable factors is then much higher.

Activity 1.2:   Stages in the planning process

1   If you were going to pre-plan a health communication campaign to promote the wearing of a seatbelt in a car, what key planning steps would you need to include? Think broadly from the conception of the campaign to the very end of the campaign.

Planning models typically follow a series of steps in a logical order. These sequential steps vary somewhat between different planning models. McKenzie et al. (2005) propose that these steps are: understanding and engaging, assessing needs, setting goals and objectives, developing a campaign, implementing the campaign and evaluating the campaign. Other common steps in a planning model include examining the evidence base, identifying budget and resources and identifying methods. The steps included in planning models are usually represented in diagrammatic forms – usually circular or linear – to enable the health practitioner to work towards their desired outcomes.

CHOOSING A MODEL

In small-scale campaigns a basic planning model will suffice. Practitioners can then choose to add other planning tools (see Chapters 2 and 3) to their own campaign plans. Larger-scale projects, especially if they involve more than a small group of people and have larger budgets, stakeholders or target groups, may find that the more complex planning models provide scope for this level of attention to detail. Generally, the bigger the project, the more factors need to be accounted for and therefore more pre-planning is required.

Selection of a planning model is not merely a matter of personal preference. McKenzie et al. (2005) highlight a number of reasons for the choice of a planning model including the preference of stakeholders and the time available for the planning process. A wide range of planning models are used in health promotion and public health practice. The further reading at the end of this chapter indicates where you can find information about additional models not covered this textbook. In this chapter we consider four planning models that can be used for health communication campaigns. They are:

1   The nine-step planning model.
2   Total Process Planning Model (National Social Marketing Council 2006b).
3   PRECEDE–PROCEED (Green and Kreuter 2005).
4   Intervention Mapping (Bartholomew et al. 2006).

The first two of these are sequential planning models incorporating basic stage/step models of planning. They are less complex than some other planning models as they follow a logical sequence and allow room for additional variables to be included as necessary.

The more complex planning models considered in this chapter are the *PRECEDE-PROCEED* model and *Intervention Mapping* (IM). These models are more rigid and prescriptive in nature. While there are a number of other planning models available to practitioners (some of which use computer-based software), these two models are commonly used in health and have demonstrated their use in a range of health promotion and public health-based work, showing adaptability to health campaigns.

THE NINE-STEP MODEL

The nine-step model is cyclical in form. It is based on the idea that feedback from one campaign can contribute to the development of the next. The steps in the nine-step model (see Figure 1.1) are (1) Rationale, needs and priorities (2) Aims and objectives (3) Selection of theoretical model (4) Method and design of method (5) Resources/budget (6) Evaluation (7) Action plan (8) Implementation and (9) Feedback and future. Each step will be described in turn.

Step 1:   Rationale: the rationale is written, including the evidence base to identify the main reasons for the campaign. Needs and priorities are also decided.
Step 2:   Aims and objectives: this is where aims and objectives are set.
Step 3:   Selection of theoretical model: a theoretical model is selected to provide the basis for the campaign.
Step 4:   Method and design of method: the method and how the method will be designed are formulated here. The method is *what* will be done, and the design is *how* this will be done.

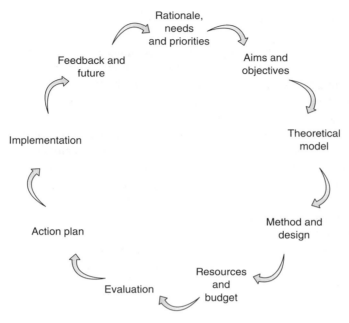

Figure 1.1   Nine-step planning model

Step 5:   Resources and budget: this is a list of resources, and a matching list of how much these resources will cost, including manpower, practical resources and other factors that might involve financial or resource issues.

Step 6:   Evaluation: this indicates the evaluation method and how this will be conducted.

Step 7:   Action plan: this is a full action plan detailing what will happen and when.

Step 8:   Implementation: this stage is devoted to the full implementation of the campaign.

Step 9:   Feedback: this is the feedback of evaluation results and campaign developments. This also includes recommendations that can be used for future evidence-based practice.

As a straightforward model, the nine-step model is suitable for most small-scale campaigns. This includes those campaigns that are running on a small budget or a limited time scale.

Activity 1.3:   Planning using the nine-step model

You are designing a campaign to promote oral hygiene in the under-fives in your local area, and you want to develop an oral health pack for parents/carers. Your overall aim is 'to increase the number of parents who brush their children's teeth correctly for three minutes at least once a day'. You have £1000 to help you run your campaign.

1   Using the nine-step model, plan a campaign based on this topic that is within this budget. Remember that you will need to formulate objectives, identify all the resources you will need, and think about how you will evaluate your work.

TOTAL PROCESS PLANNING

Social marketing can be used to help the campaign planning process. Social marketing applied to health involves 'the systematic application of marketing concepts and techniques to achieve specific behaviour goals relevant to improving health and reducing health *inequalities*' (NSMC 2006b). The frameworks and principles that social marketing embodies have been found to be useful in a variety of health contexts, and therefore can be fully integrated into a range of health-related communication campaigns (Corcoran 2008). Social marketing follows a clear framework and this makes it easier to identify the factors that influence behaviour (Corcoran 2007a). Social marketing has been used recently in a number of health areas including physical activity (Dearing et al. 2006; Gordon et al. 2006) and HIV/AIDS (Lombardo and Leger 2007).

The National Social Marketing Council (NSMC) (2006a) argues that the planning process should be systematic. In particular, it advocates that attention should be given to 'scoping and development'. The NSMC recommend a model entitled 'the Total Process Planning' model (TPP). This five-step model is illustrated in Figure 1.2. The five steps (or phases) in the model are: (1) scope; (2) develop; (3) implement; (4) evaluate; and (5) follow-up.

The five steps

1 Scope

The scoping phase examines and defines the key issue(s) of the campaign. This includes clarifying aims, segmenting the audience, identifying the behavioural focus and engaging stakeholders. Therefore the main focus in this section is examining and defining the issues (with stakeholders), reviewing the focus of the audience, focusing attention on the specific targeted behaviours and establishing goals. Finally, development of the proposition (similar to the main messages) will be completed at this stage.

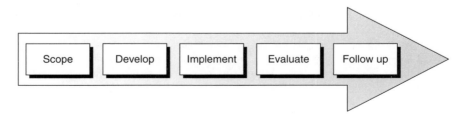

Figure 1.2   Total Process Planning model

Source: Adapted from National Social Marketing Council (2006a).

Case study 1.1:   Collecting data in the scoping phase

Duyn et al. (2007) indicate there are two ways to ensure that evidence is sufficient to inform a social marketing campaign. The first way is to segment the target audience and then examine what appeals to that audience. The second is to use 'gatekeepers' (those people who influence the target population) to learn about aspects of the target group, for example, traditionally held example beliefs. This might involve focus groups, surveys, questionnaires, examining popular media or literature or other methods.

2 Develop

In the development phase, the campaign proposition is tested and a plan for action is developed. Activities include selecting the appropriate social marketing activities, pre-testing materials, and defining appropriate indicators for evaluation. Pre-testing and re-testing the proposition will take place here also so that the campaign is ready for the next phase.

This phase employs a well-known concept called the 'marketing mix'. This consists of what have become known as 'the four Ps', namely:

- Product
- Price
- Place
- Promotion/positioning.

'Product' refers to the characteristics of the product itself. Price is the cost (not just actual costs, but imagined costs too). Place is where the product (or behaviour) is available, e.g. community centres. Promotion/positioning is the way in which the product is sold. This includes the publicity and message design associated with the 'product'.

The 'price' of a campaign does not always refer to actual price in money: it may include psychological or social prices. For example, buying a packet of condoms is generally regarded as a monetary price. However, the secondary behaviour (using the condoms) is actually what may elicit higher costs, as negotiating safer sex may actually come at a high price. This may include embarrassment or being seen as promiscuous, for suggesting condoms are used. In a marital relationship there may also be different 'costs' in asking for a condom, such as being labelled as unfaithful.

Activity 1.4:   Designing campaigns using the 4 Ps

You are undertaking a campaign to encourage girls aged 11–13 to become more physically active after school. After focus groups with groups of 11–13-year-olds you find two main areas of interest. First, girls do not want to spend 'pocket' money on

(Continued)

(*Continued*)

physical activities, and, second, they say they do not have time in their school week to exercise due to extra-curricular groups, homework and socializing. You have been allocated some money for resources, and are planning to promote different ways to be active in the local park promoted through a small fold-out booklet.

1 Based on the information above what is your: Product? Price? Place? and Promotion?

3 Implement
The implementation phase involves the commencement and management of the actual campaign.

4 Evaluate
In this phase the campaign processes, the outcomes of the campaign, and its cost effectiveness are evaluated. The actual impact on the goals therefore should be identified through this process.

5 Follow up
The follow-up phase consists of capitalizing on the successes of the campaign, constructing a review, and recording information for future reference, for example in subsequent campaigns. The model emphasizes the strong involvement of stakeholders throughout the planning process.

The social marketing approach has been subject to a number of criticisms (see Corcoran 2007a). In relation to its use as a planning model, however, Lombardo and Leger (2007) note that in their review of two HIV/AIDS campaign that used social marketing principles, behavioural models of health were not included in the social marketing campaigns. This may be a problematic area of social marketing as it does not explicitly include a section to incorporate relevant behavioural change theories, unlike the other planning models discussed. In addition, the other criticisms of social marketing in general, such as ignoring wider structural barriers to change by putting emphasis on individuals (Lombardo and Leger 2007), may also apply to the use of social marketing as a planning model. More information on the use of social marketing in health communication is given in Chapter 5.

PRECEDE–PROCEED MODEL

The PRECEDE–PROCEED model (Green and Kreuter 2005) is widely known. As shown in Figure 1.3, it comprises nine steps. 'PRECEDE' stands for 'Predisposing, Reinforcing and Enabling Constructs in Educational/Ecological Diagnosis and Evaluation' (Green and Kreuter 2005). The model 'provides a

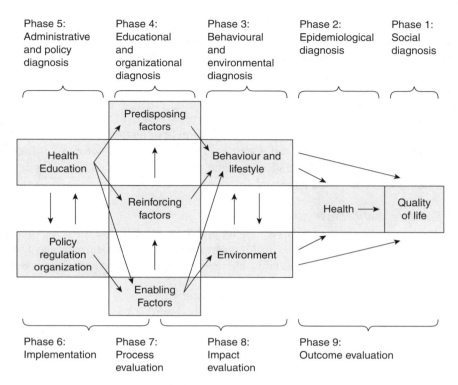

Figure 1.3   PRECEDE–PROCEED planning model
Source: Adapted from Green and Kreuter (2005).

clear systematic process for planning, delivering, and evaluating health promotion campaigns for defined populations' (Meador and Linnan 2006: 187). The model has been widely used in health promotion and health education and is grounded theory, as well as providing a comprehensive planning model (McKenzie et al. 2005). It has been developed and adapted over time with the addition recently of 'PROCEED' to the framework. PROCEED stands for 'Policy, Regulatory and Organizational Constructs in Educational and Environmental Development'.

Many campaigns have utilized the PRECEDE model. Most recently these include planning campaigns concerning men's health (Meador and Linnan 2006), mental health promotion (Mo and Mak 2008), early psychosis (Yeo et al. 2007), and cardiovascular disease (Ramey et al. 2008).

Although this model may look complicated, it is actually one of the most straightforward planning models. PRECEDE starts with the desired outcome and then works backwards systematically to complete a campaign plan. Generally the premise of the model is that the PRECEDE phase uses data and information from the early stages to create an educational and ecological assessment of the problem (Ramey et al. 2008). The PROCEED phase then guides the evaluation process. PRECEDE can be used without the PROCEED elements, and practitioners may wish either to use the two elements together, or to choose only the first, depending on campaign design.

The stages

1 Social assessment

This stage involves the identification of the target population's concerns, needs and quality of life, problems and priorities. This section could compose of focus groups, interviews, surveys and systematic searching of the wider issues connected with the proposed target group.

2 Epidemiological assessment

In this stage, data is used to prioritize the problems identified in Stage 1. This is generally a case of ranking the health issues from most to least important. Data may include morbidity and mortality, alongside markers such as prevalence rates.

3 Behavioural and environmental assessment

In this stage the key behavioural and environmental factors associated with the health problem(s) identified in Stage 2 are established. Behavioural factors therefore may include preventative behaviours, fitness levels, etc. Environmental factors will include the wider environment, for example, accessible services or affordability.

Activity 1.5:   What factors are important in Stage 3?

Wasilewski et al. (2008) examined the prevention of work-related musculoskeletal disorders in supermarket cashiers. They list a number of behavioural and environmental determinants that could contribute to musculoskeletal disorders. They also include a third factor. This is 'rehabilitation factors' such as biomechanical and functional status as they contribute to work-related injuries. The rehabilitation factors specific to the supermarket cashier group included decreased muscular endurance (from inactivity), and repetitive movement (from scanning).

1 If you were conducting the same study on supermarket cashiers, which behavioural and environmental determinants (part of the Stage 3 assessment) do you think contribute to musculoskeletal disorders such as back pain? Use the stage explanations to help you.
2 Based on your answer to the above, what sort of messages might you include in a campaign to address these determinants?

---

4 Educational and ecological assessment

In this stage, the factors that may influence behaviour are identified. These are split into pre-disposing, enabling and reinforcing factors. *Predisposing factors* include a person's *attitudes*, *beliefs* and *values*. *Enabling factors* include resources available and the skills necessary for change. *Reinforcing factors* denote feedback received by significant others, friends, peers, family that may act as barriers to change or support benefits.

5 Administrative and policy assessment

In this stage we determine the capabilities and resources available to develop and implement the campaign. This includes, for example, organizational capacity, or current policies. Yeo et al. (2007) describe an early diagnosis psychosis public education campaign where they identify that open-referral policies from the wider community (for example, educational establishments or friends) are better for facilitating early diagnosis than those that rely on referrals purely from the medical profession, highlighting how policies may be influential in campaign development.

Stages 6 to 9

With Stage 6 we shift from the PRECEDE model to the PROCEED model.

Stage 6: Implementation.

Stages 7 to 9: Process, impact and outcome evaluation.

These variables are considered in more detail in subsequent chapters.

Case study 1.2:   Predisposing, Enabling and Reinforcing in mental health promotion

Mo and Mak (2008) undertook a study using PRECEDE to help understand mental health-promoting behaviours in Hong Kong. They highlight the role of predisposing, enabling and reinforcing factors as antecedents to behaviour change. Mo and Mak explain that *Predisposing factors* are individual characteristics (i.e. attitudes, beliefs). *Enabling factors* are objective aspects linked to the individual that are objective, i.e. skills, wider environment. *Reinforcing factors* are the perceived benefits, barriers, rewards, or punishments as a consequence of performing that behaviour. In relation to mental health, *'sense of coherence'* was seen as a predisposing factor, *'daily hassles'* as an enabling factor, and *'social support'* as a reinforcing factor. They proposed that these factors would act as antecedents to mental health-promoting behaviours. Their study found that all of these were significantly linked to mental health-promoting behaviours. This illustrates the importance of identifying predisposing, enabling and reinforcing factors in Stage 4 which could provide a basis for campaign messages.

INTERVENTION MAPPING (IM)

IM is 'a stepwise approach for theory and evidence based development and implementation of campaigns' (Wolfers et al. 2007: 142). It can be used to aid campaign planners to make appropriate decisions during the development of a campaign (Reinaerts et al. 2008). The IM model provides a 'common creative framework' (Aarø et al. 2006: 152) which allows health practitioners to include key aspects of the planning process in their work, ensure their work is evidence-based, and include both participants and other stakeholders in the planning process. Thus, IM proposes a path to follow from the identification of a problem to the proposal of a solution (Kok et al. 2004).

IM offers several benefits. Not only does it ensure that the evidence base is used, but also that clear objectives are set and theoretical models incorporated into health-related campaigns. The IM also offers a perspective that includes the wider factors that influence health, often referred to as the ecological approach. This approach recognises that behaviour is influenced by factors such as intra-personal, cultural factors and the wider physical environment (Reinaerts et al. 2008). Thus, the model acknowledges that health is linked both to individuals and their environment (Aarø et al. 2006), and distinguishes between individual and environmental determinants (Brug et al. 2005). The model has not just been used for new campaigns, but also in the adaptation of existing campaigns to practice (Tortolero et al. 2005).

IM has been used in the health field in a wide range of areas. In recent years IM has been applied to areas such as sexual health (Wolfers et al. 2007; Aarø et al. 2006), healthy lifestyles (Heinen et al. 2006), worksite physical activity (McEachan et al. 2008), behaviour nutrition and physical activity (Brug et al. 2005), and fruit and vegetable consumption (Reinaerts et al. 2008).

Initially IM comprised five stages (Bartholomew et al. 2001). This was later extended to six to include the needs assessment stage considered important to the planning process (Bartholomew et al. 2006). The six stages are shown in Figure 1.4.

The stages

1 Needs assessment
This stage involves identification of the problem on which the campaign will focus and examination of the factors that contribute to the problem. There are generally two phases in the needs assessment. First, consultation with the target group via questionnaires, focus groups, interview or other methods can assist in determining aspects of the problem. This also includes identifying key behavioural and environmental determinants, for example, attitudes, beliefs, *values*, barriers and benefits.

Second, a scoping exercise to identify the scale and breadth of the issue might be used alongside analysis of the evidence base which assists in the development of a systematic review of the literature. Areas such as behavioural factors and environmental determinants are also investigated and determined alongside the main health issues connected with the problem. This process may see the emergence of themes that the campaign will centre on, and at the end of this section overall campaign outcomes based on the information from this step (see case study 1.3).

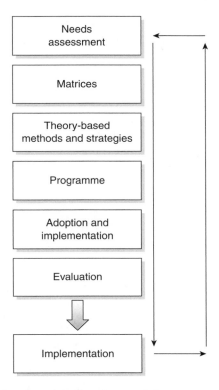

Figure 1.4   Intervention Mapping planning model
Source: Adapted from Bartholomew et al. (2006).

Case study 1.3:   IM and step 1 – needs assessment

McEachan et al. (2008) used IM to develop a worksite intervention. They used focus groups in their needs assessment section, and part of the information from the focus group was used to split information into barriers and facilitators of engaging in physical activity.

Two of the most frequently cited barriers were 'I don't have any time', and 'I am too tired by the time I finish work'. Two of the most frequently cited facilitators were 'doing things with other people' and 'having access to gym at work'. These barriers/facilitators were then used in the writing of outcomes and objectives that informed the development of the intervention.

2 Matrices

In this stage we identify who and what will change as the result of the planned campaign. This is where further clarification of the objectives is made, and the outcomes are broken down into smaller objectives called performance objectives. The determinants of behaviour that are the most important are included here.

The matrices themselves fall outside the coverage of this textbook as they are extensive. See Bartholomew et al. (2006) for more information on the matrices.

3 Theory-based methods and practical strategies

In this stage the most appropriate theoretical model is selected. This could be any of the behavioural change models (see Chapter 3), or other theoretical models that link to aspects of behavioural change. This is an important stage as theories are essential to effective campaigns (Kok et al. 2004). The practical strategies include identifying the method, strategy and materials needed. This might also include producing and pilot testing materials and defining campaign structures. Chapter 5 has more information on the design of materials.

Case study 1.4:   Choosing appropriate theories and models

Choosing a model, therefore, is based on a series of factors, and the theoretical model will vary depending on the behaviour that is highlighted.

For example Aarø et al. (2006) in their examination of the promotion of sexual and reproductive health in South Africa and Tanzania in 12–14-year-olds relied on two theoretical models: the *Theory of Planned Behaviour* (Ajzen 1991) and *Social Cognitive Theory* (Bandura 1988) – the rationale being that they both contain variables that have been linked to sexual health in a variety of studies, especially the promotion of condom use. Factors such as behavioural intentions were seen as important predictors of behaviour based on the theoretical models selected.

Hou et al. (2004), in their study of the development of a cervical cancer educational campaign for Chinese women, chose different variables from a selection of theoretical models. These included knowledge, pros and cons from the *Transtheoretical Model* (Prochaska and Diclemente 1983) and perceived susceptibility and cues to action from the *Health Belief Model* (Becker 1974).

4 Campaign

In this stage the actual campaign is designed. This includes the schedule or time-table of events, staff and stakeholder roles, how aspects of the campaign are delivered, and so on.

Activity 1.6:   Methods, strategies and materials

You are working to encourage adherence to healthy lifestyles in a group of leg ulcer patients. This group say that they believe physical activity will be uncomfortable, costly and difficult to access. This means that beliefs about physical activity are a strong determinant in this group.

1   What methods, strategies, and materials might you use to address this determinant? Remember, your method is what you will do and your strategies are how you will deliver the method. The materials are what you will need to help you deliver the strategy.

5 Adoption and implementation plan

In this stage plans for adoption and implementation are developed.

6 Evaluation plan

In this stage the plan for evaluation is developed. Ideally each campaign outcome and the performance objectives are evaluated to see if they were successfully achieved. This can be through process, impact, outcome evaluation, or cost effectiveness evaluations (see Chapter 7).

There have been some criticisms of the IM process. These include reference to the protocol being time-consuming as there is a requirement for lengthy attention to each section, particularly the matrices which can result in a huge amount of data (McEachan et al. 2008). In addition, the complexity of this model may mean that health practitioners who are not specifically trained in planning models may find the stages difficult without additional training and guidance. In addition, there is a possibility that the rigid nature of this model may allow less room for more creative communication strategies.

PRINCIPLES AND VALUES

The main criticism of the current planning models is that they exclude traditional health promotion principles and values. This is of particular concern to those practitioners who feel that values and principles are an important part of the planning process. Gregg and O'Hara (2007) note that planning models used in health are often technical in nature as their focus follows systematic steps in the planning process. The values and the principles that underlie action are not explicitly included. Gregg and O'Hara therefore propose an alternative planning model, entitled the 'red lotus' health promotion model, which includes the basic planning steps in 'petal layers', while ensuring sustainability, values and principles through the 'roots and leaves' of the model.

Another model that also includes values, goals and ethics is the IDM (Interactive Domain Approach Model) (Kahan and Goodstadt 2002). Although neither of these models are widely used in published research at present, they both have potential for campaigns that require a more sensitive focus, or that have a strong principles and values framework underlying the main health issue.

CHAPTER REVIEW

Planning is integral to successful campaigns. It can ensure that problems are resolved, approaches, resources and outcomes are achieved as practitioners intended and that time, money and resources are utilized effectively. There are a number of planning models available that can assist in the planning of campaigns drawn from existing health promotion and public health disciplines. Practitioners usually have only one opportunity to implement a campaign and by spending time planning first, they can ensure that this opportunity is used as effectively as possible.

This chapter has:

- explored the role of planning to ensure that campaigns have a higher success rate and limit error;
- identified a selection of planning models and considered their application to a variety of campaigns;
- examined the criticisms of these planning models and provided possible solutions or alternatives to these.

FURTHER READING

Bartholomew, L K, Parcel, G S, Kok, G and Gottlieb, N H (2006) *Planning health promotion campaigns: a campaign mapping approach*. Jossey-Bass, San Francisco.

Earle, S, Lloyd, C, Sidell, M and Spurr, S (2007) *Theory and research in promoting public health*. Sage/The Open University, London.

Green, L W and Kreuter, M W (2005) *Health promotion planning: an educational and ecological approach*, *3rd edition*. McGraw-Hill, Maidenhead.

2

Frameworks and foundations

This chapter outlines the frameworks and foundations needed to construct successful campaigns. This includes a focus on setting aims and objectives, deciding on appropriate methods, identifying stakeholders and decision-makers, and selecting and incorporating appropriate theoretical models. This chapter identifies three theoretical models and analyses their application to practice in the design of health campaigns.

This chapter aims to:

- identify ways to set SMART aims and objectives
- examine appropriate methodologies
- analyse the role of stakeholders and decision-makers and consider ways to include these in campaigns
- identify and incorporate theoretical models into practice

AIMS AND OBJECTIVES

The developmental phase of a campaign centres on: (1) constructing suitable aims and objectives; (2) selecting an appropriate theoretical basis; and (3) examining methodologies. Subsequently this process needs to take into account a wide range of factors including the planning model used (as discussed in Chapter 1) and clear identification of target groups, health issues, and locations (see Chapter 3). Bos et al. propose that the planning stage means practitioners can acknowledge the role of 'environments, including families, social networks, organizations, and public policy frameworks' (2008: 451).

A major phase in the design of campaigns is the formulation of aims and objectives. Every planned and well-constructed campaign has a way of defining what it wants to achieve and all campaigns will generally have one or two aims and a number of objectives. Some campaigns may also have a goal (see below). For the purposes of this textbook we will assume the following terminology:

- Goal: what a campaign intends to achieve overall, usually in the wider arena of health.
- Aim: what a campaign aims to achieve overall.
- Objectives: a specific statement that indicates how the aim will be achieved.

An aim is what you want the campaign to achieve, for example, an increase or decrease in a behaviour. The objectives specify how the aim will be achieved, for example, through increasing skills or challenging beliefs. Larger campaigns may also have a goal. A goal is the wider target that is trying to be achieved, for example, the overall goal of a campaign might be to reduce childhood hospital admissions, but the aim of the campaign is to reduce rates of measles in under-fives through increasing vaccinate uptake, which could lead to a reduction in hospital admissions.

Case study 2.1: Setting goals and objectives in 'Camine Con Nosotros'

Soto Mas et al. (2000) report on the design of Camine Con Nosotros (come walk with us). The overall goal is to decrease risk factors for cardiovascular disease by increasing participants' physical activity levels. They set campaign requirements to help to identify the target group (low-income women from underserved communities and a high number of Mexican-descent Hispanics).

The programme used focus groups and a literature review to help decide objectives and methods. For example, the literature review established that low to moderate intensity exercise based in the home was more likely to be adopted, as well as walking being a preferred means of activity. Walking is also considered appropriate for a group who may have limited access to resources. Therefore, objectives were formulated around moderate level physical activity following the current recommendations of five times of 30 minutes a week.

A well-designed campaign always has objectives. These are the main elements that will be measured to ensure the campaign is successful (see Chapter 7 for more on evaluation). Soto Mas et al. (2000) suggest that the identification of goals and objectives should take place prior to selection of the theoretical framework. A chosen aim will also dictate which methods are the most appropriate. For example, an aim to raise awareness will have a different method from one that intends to change a factor in the social environment. Objectives can be challenging to formulate. There is no room for inaccuracies when setting objectives. Poor objectives usually mean a campaign cannot achieve its aim. If objectives are not achieved, then often the aim will not be achieved.

Objectives usually include an 'active' phrase, suggesting that objectives are something that will be 'undertaken'. Examples of such phrases include 'to increase …' 'to raise awareness of …' and 'to identify …'. Table 2.1 lists the types of objectives and possible definitions of these. Different objectives use different terminology, for example, a behavioural objective will be centred on being able to do something and therefore to demonstrate or perform, whereas a knowledge objective will be centred on memory and words such as recall or identify.

Table 2.1 Example words that can be used when formulating objectives

Type of objective	Example words	Examples in practice
Knowledge objective	– Describe – Outline – Identify – Explain – Design – Recall – Demonstrate	'Explain the three main elements of the Green Cross Code' 'Recall two safe places to cross the road'
Attitudinal objective	– Demonstrate – Recognize – Be able to – Identify – Utilize – Show – Formulate	'Demonstrate the ability to use pedestrian crossings in the face of peer opposition' 'Formulate responses to peers when challenged on the wearing of a seatbelt'
Behavioural objective	– Perform – Observe – Describe – Demonstrate – Undertake – Be able to – Apply	'Demonstrate the ability to cross the road safely at a pedestrian crossing' 'Apply the Green Cross Code to a real traffic situation'

Activity 2.1:   Formulating different objectives

You are working on a campaign to increase awareness of triggers for asthma in households with one asthmatic child. You also want to encourage family members to change their behaviour accordingly (for example, not smoking indoors).

1 Formulate three objectives (one knowledge, one behaviour and one attitude) that could be objectives in this campaign. Use Table 2.1 to help you.

A campaign's objectives should be SMART. There are variations as to what SMART means but here it is used to mean the following:

Specific: This means your objective needs to be a specific statement that clearly states its purpose.
Measurable: This means your objective can be measured though the evaluation process.
Achievable: This means your objective needs to be able to be achieved by your target group.

Realistic: This means your objective needs to have a realistic outcomes.
Timebound: This means your objective needs to be set to a specific timeframe in order for it to be measured.

A campaign may have a number of objectives. There are a range of different variables that you might want to try and manipulate or change. For example, objectives could be linked to recall of information or demonstration knowledge. These would require different objectives. Unless you are working on a very large campaign, you will generally not have more than four or five objectives. Any more than this will mean that your project may be too complex and difficult to evaluate. These objectives may all be centred on one area (for example, all knowledge objectives), but often they will relate to a combination of knowledge, attitude or behaviour.

Activity 2.2:   Matching objectives to your aim

You are working in a local hospital to reduce MRSA (Methicillin-resistant Staphylococcus aureus). The campaign has a range of posters in strategic locations around the hospital and ensures that bacterial hand gel dispensers are located at the entrance/exit to every ward.

Aim: To reduce the incidence of MRSA within a hospital ward within a six-month period.
Objective 1: To increase by 50 per cent the number of visitors who use anti-bacterial hand gel dispensers before entering and exiting a ward.

1   What other SMART objectives could you have that would ensure you achieve your aim?

MATCHING AIMS WITH METHODS

One of the difficulties with aims and objectives is matching them to the appropriate methods and channels of communication. Channels of communication refer to the main types of media used (for example, television, leaflets, face-to-face). The method is how these channels are used (for example, the actual design of a television drama). Different objectives rely on different channels and different methods. For example, an objective that is centred on changing behaviour would not rely on awareness raising through leaflets to change behaviour as this is unlikely to achieve the objective. Research by Hill and Abraham (2008) notes that condom promotion leaflets can alter some cognitive antecedents but not increase use of condoms. This example illustrates that although there may be some increases in other variables, behaviour is not one of these.

An objective that intended to increase knowledge might use leaflets, but one that wants to change behaviour would use additional methods. Using more than one method is often advised in campaigns as good practice (see, for example,

Table 2.2 Five objectives and their application to methods

Type of objective	Example words for objectives	Example communication channels	Example objective and method
Awareness	To raise awareness of … To increase awareness of …	Exhibitions Mass media methods: leaflets, posters, flyers, video, television, radio	**Aim:** To raise awareness of National No Smoking Day **Method:** A stop smoking exhibition stand
Knowledge	To increase knowledge of … To increase the number of people who can …	Mass media methods: leaflets, posters, flyers, television, radio and written materials One-to-one or small group teaching	**Aim:** To increase the number of people in a workplace who can list four ways to reduce their cholesterol levels **Method:** A short five-minute group talk in team meetings
Attitudinal	To promote more positive attitudes towards … To reduce negative attitudes towards …	Skills-based training workshops/programs Small group work Role-play	**Aim:** To increase the number of 15-year-olds at a youth centre who have positive attitudes towards condom purchase **Method:** Role-play-based activities
Empowerment	To enable a group of people to … To increase the number of people who can …	Skills training, small group work, peer education, demonstration, written material	**Aim:** To increase the number of people who can cook one healthy meal a week for their family **Method**: Skills-based half-day workshop
Behaviour	To increase the number of people who can … To reduce the number of people who …	Interactive workshops or training programs Possible 'trigger' points based on theoretical models	**Aim:** To increase the number of students who live in a two-mile radius of a university to walk to the campus once a week. **Method:** Incentive-based free, interactive physical activity workshops

Corcoran 2007a; Heitzler et al. 2008; Hoa et al. 2009). Chapter 5 also discusses this in more detail. Methods therefore have to be matched to objectives. Table 2.2 illustrates the possible types of campaign objectives, channels of communication, and the possible methods that could be used in campaigns that match these.

Table 2.2 uses five popular objectives: (1) awareness; (2) knowledge; (3) attitudinal; (4) empowerment; and (5) behavioural objectives. It then gives examples of possible channels of communication that could be used as well as an example method for each type of objective. An objective will usually fit into one (or possibly two) of the categories in Table 2.2. Any more than this and the objective is probably too broad and may need refining. An exception is very large-scale campaigns that may incorporate a wide range of factors. If this is the case, some methods do span more than one aim, so it may be possible to choose one or two methods that cover all of these areas.

Activity 2.3:   Which methods best suit which objectives?

1 Read the aims below and using Table 2.2 identify which each one is (awareness, knowledge, attitudinal, empowerment, behavioural).
2 What types of channels of communication could you use, and what type of methods?

   (i)   To increase the number of children aged 6–8 washing their hands before eating food in a school by 30 per cent.
   (ii) To increase the number of older adults in a day centre able to recall three possible signs of diabetes.

DECISION-MAKERS AND STAKEHOLDERS

Decision-makers and stakeholders are key people in the campaign process. Not only should they be involved in the formulation of aims and objectives, they should be key participants in the subsequent planning process. Collaboration with target groups, decision-makers and stakeholders is important to 'identify the optimal intervention' (Bos et al. 2008: 451). Close collaboration with these groups can ensure campaigns are likely to be more successful. Campaigns may also have 'partnerships', which in some cases may replace stakeholders. Goldman and Schmalz (2007) propose a series of principles of partnerships that can be applied to the context of stakeholders as well as partnerships. They propose reasons for partnering, including access to more resources and shared ownership. Benefits of partnering include increasing credibility and minimizing duplication.

Campaigns vary in their stakeholders. An intervention that encourages physical activity using after-school clubs would have different stakeholders than a campaign intending to increase vigilance of theft in local pubs and bars. Brown et al. (2006) note that informants in a rapid appraisal in a community setting included a voluntary worker, a Sister from the Catholic Church, counsellors, the project coordinators, local police, a pharmacist, head teachers, a shopkeeper, a local health visitor, and a housing department officer.

Activity 2.4:   Choosing stakeholders

1 Identify which stakeholders you would include in the campaigns below. Assume that these campaigns would all be undertaken in your local area. Consider at least 10 people/groups/organizations you could include for each.

   (i)   Aim: To increase knowledge in supermarket shoppers of a food traffic light system (red = high in fat, green = low in fat) in a supermarket.
   (ii) Aim: To increase knowledge in young people aged 16–20 in a large factory setting of modes of transmission of HIV/AIDS and risks to their own health.

Cameron et al. (2008) indicate that as health becomes more holistic in nature, so the number of stakeholders increases. They note that each stakeholder comes with their own perspective and understandings as to what health is. This may then impact on what they do and say in the project.

In some campaigns, private organizations and businesses may be as important as public sector organizations. Health is not just an issue for those who work in health. For example, Activity 2.4 would probably identify local authorities, supermarkets and factory owners as part of the stakeholder list. Involvement in health-related projects depends on a number of factors including the health issue, location, interest, resources, and importance. A health stand, located in a shopping centre, dealing with healthy eating might want to involve local food producers. Similarly a podiatry stand on healthy feet might want to involve pharmacists or shoe retailers. In addition, some campaign methods such as media advocacy will need to involve private organizations. Utzinger et al. (2004) in their study on a community outreach programme in Chad-Cameroon use a high level of public–private partnerships. They note with increasing globalization that capacities of governments have diminished and private enterprises may be seen as more powerful in achieving change. This is particularly of note in developing countries where there may be shortages of resources and health personnel. It is also worth noting that stakeholders can be problematic as they may have differing agendas.

Case study 2.2: Influences on sexual health education

Research by Bosmans et al. (2006) in the Democratic Republic of Congo (DRC) centred on adolescent sexual health programmes and problems accessing sexual health-related information. Because the DRC is an area with poor health infrastructures and systems, sexual health education has predominantly been delivered by organizations which are heavily influenced by the Catholic Church. These restrictions and interpretations of what the Catholic Church says on sexual health education were found to be considerable barriers to sexual health education. This includes reducing the traditional ABC approach (abstinence, being faithful, condom use), to AB (i.e. removing condom use from the formula) and thus abstinence was promoted as the only responsible way of behaving.

The article suggests that instead of concluding that Catholic organizations should not be allowed to deliver sexual and reproductive health programmes, it is actually of great importance to include them in any programme. This will then mean that the gap between socio-cultural religious values and adolescents' own rights to sexuality education can be addressed. Only then can information that is accurate and free of any norms or bias be achievable.

A number of questions need to be considered when identifying stakeholders. These include who will be involved, and what their main roles will be. Additional considerations include the questions of how feedback will be disseminated between stakeholders and which mechanisms will be used. Steering groups, for example, are common in campaigns to assist with this process.

THEORETICAL MODELS

The next step is to consider which theoretical model to adopt. This is essential in any campaign where the overarching aim is to result in a change in behaviour. The process of selecting a theoretical model can mean juggling aims, objectives and methods to ensure that your campaign design is appropriate.

Considerable research indicates that theoretical models are important in campaign design. Essentially health behaviour theories are an explicit statement of which processes are hypothesized to regulate behaviour (Rothman 2004). Theories can help practitioners understand the complexities of behaviour and information development and implementation of campaigns by appraising problems and identifying factors to modify (Green 2000). Theory also helps in the identification of outcomes (Bos et al. 2008). Theories and models cannot guarantee campaign success but they do provide a framework that can guide practitioners (Soto Mas et al. 2000).

Theories should form the basis for the design process in any communication intervention. Tufano and Karras (2005) indicate that by selecting key design features from theoretical models the likelihood of promoting and sustaining a behaviour change is higher. In addition, Lyles et al. (2007) note, in relation to effective HIV behaviours in at-risk populations, all the best evidence interventions rely on at least one behaviour change theory or model. Noar et al. (2009) also note the increasing success of campaigns that contain theoretically based behaviour change elements.

Although the application of theory is recommended, practitioners may find it difficult to connect theory to practice. This is partly because of the number of decision points that face practitioners at each stage of intervention development (Fishbein and Cappella 2006). As a consequence, theoretical models in health interventions can easily be overlooked (Whittingham et al. 2008). There are also gaps in the understanding of health behaviour change (Rothman 2004) and many research articles promote the use of theory but are unable to guide the practitioner in their practical application. Green (2000) also notes that lack of guidelines on selection of which theory to use and little guidance on the rationale for selection of different theories are also problematic. There is also little research on how to turn theory into persuasive messages (Noar et al. 2009). Thus the evidence generally points to clear integration of theoretical models into communication and health practice. The question is, which theory should be used, and how can it actually be used in campaign practice?

There is a wide range of theoretical models available. Here we consider three of the most common theoretical models and give a brief description of these before analysing how they can be applied to health campaigns either in their entirety or in part through case studies, activities and examples. The three models are:

- Health Belief Model (HBM) (Becker 1974)
- Theory of Planned Behaviour (TPB) (Ajzen 1980)
- Transtheoretical Model (TTM) or Stages of Change model (Prochaska and Diclemente 1983).

THE HEALTH BELIEF MODEL

The Health Belief Model (HBM) (Becker 1974) may be used in campaigns designed to influence individual behaviour (see Figure 2.1). The model may be used to assess the likelihood of individuals adopting a health behaviour based on perceptions of risk, benefits, barriers, perceived susceptibility, and perceived severity. Thus, performing a behaviour is based on these vulnerability variables (susceptibility/severity or risk). Information is then tailored to key lever points to try and elicit change. The model also includes demographic variables and a cue to action (for example, a leaflet or advice) as a prompt for the HBM process to start.

The HBM includes four factors that need to be taken into account when trying to change a behaviour. Corcoran (2007) characterizes these as follows:

- a person needs to have an incentive to perform a behaviour;
- the person must feel there is a risk in continuing the behaviour;
- the person must feel that benefits will outweigh the barriers;
- the person must have confidence (self-efficacy) to perform that behaviour.

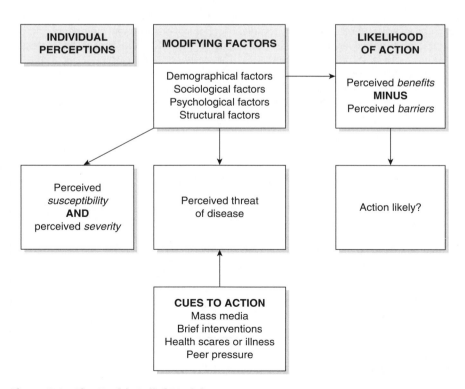

Figure 2.1   The Health Belief Model
Source: Adapted from Becker (1974).

The HBM includes variables such as risk perception, benefits, barriers, severity, and cues to action, which all can be used for targeting an intervention.

A number of recent studies have examined the role of the HBM in practice, for example, Sohl and Moyer (2007) found in a meta-analysis that mammography interventions tailored to the HBM were seen to be effective, possibly due to the nature of the model and the different types of tailoring possibilities. This is supported by Champion et al. (2008), who indicate a number of HBM variables are associated with mammography screening for African-American women. The study notes that self-efficacy and benefits were related to fear and that women who had increased perceived self-efficacy and benefits had decreased fear. In addition, HBM has recently been used in the areas of HPV vaccine acceptability (Marlow et al. 2009), mammography (Champion et al. 2008; Sohl and Moyer 2007), abstinence (Iriyama et al. 2007), calcium and exercise (Swaim et al. 2008), and condom use (Wang et al. 2009).

Case study 2.3:   Diabetes and the HBM

Gallivan et al. (2007) designed a campaign based on the HBM and the TTM (see later p.35). The campaign theme was 'Control your Diabetes. For life'. The campaign messages were framed to fit with HBM constructs and participants were seen to need to believe that the benefits of good diabetes control outweighed the risks of complications (benefits versus barriers). Constructs of the HBM were applied to the television, radio and print advertisements. The television advertisement incorporated testimonials of people with diabetes and increased perceived severity by using two characters who said "I don't want to go blind. I don't want to lose a foot or a leg. I don't want to have kidney failure." This was followed by a positive message about diabetes control.

Activity 2.5:   Using the HBM in practice

You are designing a mammography screening poster aimed specifically at West African older women (60 upwards) to promote mammography. This group live predominantly with their families and attend church frequently. You have identified that self-efficacy and the perceived benefits of screening are low in this group. Based on this information and the HBM:

1   What messages could you use for your posters to try and increase self-efficacy and the benefits of screening in this target group?
2   Where could you put your poster?

THE THEORY OF PLANNED BEHAVIOUR (TPB) MODEL

The Theory of Planned Behaviour (TPB) (Ajzen 1991) proposes that the strongest determinant of behaviour is 'behavioural intentions' (see Figure 2.2). These

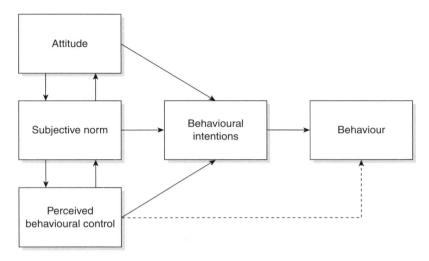

Figure 2.2   The Theory of Planned Behaviour
Source: Adapted from Ajzen (1991).

behavioural intentions are based on three factors: attitude; *subjective norm*; and   »
perceived behavioural control.   »

Attitude is related to the balance of advantages and disadvantages associated with the behaviour. In relation to tobacco smoking, people might consider many positive factors associated with smoking if they currently smoke. 'Subjective norm' refers to the influence of significant others, such as family and friends, for example, if parents or friends smoke, this may have an influence on smoking behaviours. Perceived behavioural control is the perception that a person has about their ability to perform that behaviour, for example, this could be the ability of a smoker to quit smoking.

The TPB can be used in a variety of ways in a campaign, see case study 2.4. The TPB is used extensively in health, and has been used recently to predict intentions to breast self-examine (Mason and White 2008), increase fruit and vegetable consumption (Gratton et al. 2007), increase physical activity and nutrition (Maddock et al. 2008), encourage exercise (Hill et al. 2007), condom use (Boer and Mashamba 2007), implement sun safety (White et al. 2008), testicular self-examination (McGilligan et al. 2009), and ecstasy use (Peters et al. 2007).

Case study 2.4:   TPB for leaflet design

Hill et al. (2007) used the TPB to design a leaflet to target intentions, behavioural control, attitudes, and normative beliefs in relation to energetic exercise outside Physical Education classes in adolescents. Different activities were listed alongside participants being encouraged to increase their exercise session by one week. Examples of the leaflets' messages are below:

1   To promote positive attitudes to exercise, for example, 'exercise can stop you putting on weight'.
2   To target normative beliefs by highlighting roles of significant others, for example, 'it's cool to be fit and healthy'.
3   Enhance behavioural control, for example, 'exercise such as jogging is free'.
4   Prompt daily exercise intentions, for example, 'build exercise into your daily routine'.

The TPB proposes that different behavioural intentions will lead to different behaviours. Thus, campaigns will need to be adapted according to the behavioural intentions of the person in question. Fishbein and Yzer (2003) and Fishbein and Capella (2006) take this one step further and use a 2 × 2 intention and behaviour matrix to help with this. The matrix can detail if a person has an intention but is unable to act upon it, or if they have little intention of performing the behaviour. Interventions can be tailored accordingly. For example, if someone has an intention to eat a lower fat diet, but they have barriers stopping them (e.g. lack of knowledge of ways to integrate low fat foods into their diet), then interventions can focus on skill building, or knowledge raising. If a person has not formed an intention, interventions can focus on changing or influencing attitudes, subjective norms or self-efficacy that can influence behavioural intentions.

Research has examined the role of TPB variables in predicting outcomes. Boer and Mashamba (2007) found that male attitudes to condoms and subjective norms were significantly associated with condom use; among females, attitude and self-efficacy were associated with condom use. This suggests the possibility that different TPB variables influence different target groups.

Other research also suggests this might be the case. Caperchione et al. (2008) suggest that attitude and body mass index (BMI) were the strongest predictors of physical activity. They suggest that communicating information about the risks of weight gain associated with the lack of physical activity could influence attitude change. In addition, for those who have weight management issues, providing information linked to weight management and regular physical activity may be useful in changing negative attitudes. It is hypothesized that once attitudes towards physical activity become more positive, then intention to engage in physical activity is more likely (Caperchione et al. 2008). Flisher et al. (2007) also uses the TPB in relation to attitudes (see case study 2.5).

Case study 2.5:   TPB and partner violence

Flisher et al. (2007) examined partner violence behaviours in a high school in South Africa. Using the TPB, they found that there were associations between attitudes (for example, acceptability of assault in public), general social influences (for example, most people important to you think a boy can assault a girl), outcomes expectancy (for example, partner would become more angry if I prevent him/her from assaulting you) and partner violence intentions and behaviour with partner violence among South African adolescents. The article suggests that these constructs should be targeted in interventions that aim to reduce partner violence behaviours among adolescents.

Activity 2.6: Targeting variables

You are working on a project that aims to reduce partner violence behaviours among adolescents in a secondary school. Based on the research by Flisher et al. (2007) in case study 2.5:

1 What variables would you target?
2 What messages could you formulate to address these variables in a campaign?

TRANSTHEORETICAL MODEL (TTM)

The Transtheoretical Model (TTM) (Prochaska and Diclemente 1983), also known as the Stages of Change model, proposes that, as people make a change in their behaviour, they progress through a series of stages in a cyclic manner (see Figure 2.3). This is a popular model used in health as its ease of utility appeals to practitioners. The premise of this model is based on the idea that people move through the stages of readiness. In relation to campaign design, this suggests that interventions can be targeted to different sections of the model to enable the person to move to the next stage of change.

Although originally designed for work on tobacco smoking, the TTM model has been applied to a wide range of health behaviours. These include physical

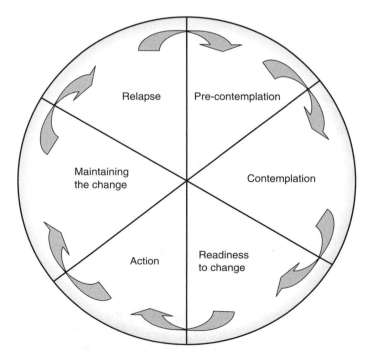

Figure 2.3   The Transtheoretical Model
Source: Adapted from Prochaska and Diclemente (1983).

activity (Dutton et al. 2008), smoking (Patten et al. 2008), healthy eating and physical activity (Johnson et al. 2008), fruit and vegetable consumption (Wiedemann et al. 2009), women at risk of HIV (Gazabon et al. 2007), bullying prevention (Evers et al. 2007), sexual health (Arden and Armitage 2008), musculoskeletal disorders (Whysall et al. 2007), and mammography (Otero-Sabogal et al. 2007).

Lowther et al. (2007) suggest that the TTM has developed four core constructs. These include the stages of change, and the processes of change, both of which are from the additional TTM model; in addition, the model also now encompasses decisional balance (i.e. pros/cons) and self-efficacy (the belief and confidence that behaviour can be changed).

Case study 2.6:   TTM and brief interventions in smoking

Patten et al. (2008) used a brief intervention for adolescent smokers. Each adolescent was assigned to a research counsellor and four factors were assessed that determined treatment content for all sessions. These were: readiness to quit smoking, social influences (for example, family and friends), psychological factors (such as coping factors), and addiction (both physical and psychological).

At each session the counsellors used motivational interviewing by focusing on a range of factors, such as reasons for change, enhancement of self-efficacy, and reinforcement of any quit attempts. Homework was given at the end of the session which focused on preparing to stop, or practising techniques discussed in the sessions. A range of materials were available to both the counsellor and adolescent, for example, on social pressure to smoking (e.g. assertiveness skills). In addition, if the adolescent was deemed to be in a preparation stage, a personal plan with a quit date and reward were drawn up.

Work by a range of authors has identified ten processes linked to specific stages of the TTM (Prochaska and Velicer 1997). These processes are emphasized at different stages of change and therefore staged matched interventions need to be matched to these ten processes. De Vet et al. (2008) successfully applied these ten stages to fruit and vegetable consumption. The stages were linked to the main TTM stages of change:

- precontemplation to contemplation; consciousness raising, dramatic relief and environmental re-evaluation;
- contemplation to preparation; self-re-evaluation;
- preparation to action; social liberation and self-liberation;
- action to maintenance; counter-conditioning, stimulus control, reinforcement management and helping relationships.

In each stage there is some particular aspect that may be targeted in an intervention, such as, in the precontemplation phase, consciousness-raising strategies might include media campaigns or feedback from health practitioners. In the preparation phase, self-re-evaluation might be altered by the use of role models. In the action/maintenance phase, stimulus control may focus on avoidance tactics, and helping relationships may employ the use of support groups.

Prochaska and Velicer (1997) suggest that, if an individual is in the precon-templation stage, consciousness-raising is important to progress to contemplation. This increases awareness about aspects of the problem such as the consequences of continuing to smoke tobacco and the availability of NRT if a person wants to make a quit attempt. In the action/maintenance stage, counter-conditioning is important for a person to move from action to maintenance. This involves the person learning a healthier behaviour to replace the problem behaviour such as coping with stress without smoking a cigarette.

Case study 2.7:   TTM and the 10 step process

Lowther et al. (2007) suggest a number of key processes associated with the TTM that can be applied to exercise behaviour change using the ten-step process. Self-liberation, for example a commitment to and a belief that the person can continue to exercise, was the most strongly associated with exercising. The article suggests therefore that the focus of an intervention that aimed to aid progression from action to maintenance could engage the participants' commitment to exercise by the rein-forcement of key messages such as the benefits of continuing regular physical activity. Self-liberation was also deemed to be important in preparation for action.

SELECTING A THEORETICAL MODEL

It can be difficult to decide which theoretical model to use. A needs assessment may identify key variables to inform this decision, or a judgement may have to be made in conjunction with a target group as to what the most important vari-ables are in relation to the health behaviours. For example, is it peer pressure that is preventing a group using condoms? The TPB might be appropriate for its inclusion of subjective norms. Is it fear of disease consequences that encourages a group to go for screening? Then HBM might be appropriate for its inclusion of perceived severity. Is it reinforcement of key healthy eating messages that encourages a target group to continue reducing their dietary fat intake? In that case, the TTM model might be appropriate for the self-liberation element in the action phase. There is not always a right and wrong model, rather it is a case of choosing a model that fits the purpose depending on circumstances.

Activity 2.7:   Matching what your target group say to theory

Look at the following examples and select which component is illustrated by the example, and which model you would then use (the components and models are listed below).

(Continued)

(Continued)

A list of components: *attitude, subjective norm, PBC, self-efficacy, susceptibility, severity, benefits, barriers, cues to action.*

A list of models: *Theory of Planned Behaviour, Health Belief Model, Transtheoretical Model.*

1 You are working on a campaign to increase testicular self-examination in adolescent boys. Their most common reasons for not undertaking self-examination are 'I am not confident enough' and 'I don't know how to do it'. Which components do these comments link to and which model could be used with this group?

2 You are working on a campaign to ensure that workers lift boxes correctly. Their most common reasons for not currently doing this are 'My chances of injuring my back are small' and 'There is only a small possibility that I will injure myself'. Which components do these comments link to and which model could be used with this group?

3 You are working on a campaign to encourage parents to reduce their children's sugar intake by half in the snacks that they provide for them. Their most common reason for not currently doing this are 'Sweet snacks are easy and keep my children quiet' and 'My children won't eat savoury snacks and complain they don't like the taste'. Which components do these comments link to and which model could be used with this group?

4 You are working on a campaign to reduce cannabis drug-driving in students. Their most common reasons for drug driving are 'My other friends do this' and 'We always do this as we need to get home'. Which components do these comments link to and which model could be used with this group?

Activity 2.7 provides an illustration of how what people say may be linked to theoretical models. This could then be used in the design of messages for your work, or in the design of resources. For example, work with example (1) from Activity 2.7, could centre on teaching the ability to self-examine, as this is the reason why this group do not currently perform the behaviour. Messages to be emphasized might be those concerning reducing barriers to self-examination and showing how self-examination can be done easily in three steps (or a similar message).

Figure 2.4 illustrates the key variables of these theoretical models. Figure 2.4 can be used to link theory to practice and may aid the selection of the appropriate theoretical model. It is important to remember though that this is just a guide and you still do need to incorporate the rest of the models' philosophies within your campaign design, for example in the design of materials (see Chapter 6).

CRITICISMS OF THEORETICAL MODELS

There have been a number of criticisms of theoretical models. These are discussed in more detail in the sources cited in the Further Reading section. It is, however, useful to mention some of the main arguments in relation to these

Variables	Health Belief Model (HBM)	Theory of Planned Behaviour (TPB)	Transtheoretical Model (TTM)
Behaviour	×		
Susceptibility	×		
Severity	×		
Threat of disease	×		
Benefits	×		
Barriers	×		
Attitude		×	
Subjective norm		×	
Perceived behavioural control		×	
Intention		×	
Pre-contemplation			×
Contemplation			×
Readiness			×
Action			×
Maintenance			×
Relapse			×
Behaviour	×	×	×

Figure 2.4 Key variables in theoretical models

models here. First, the models themselves cannot explain all behavioural outcomes; rather, they are designed as a framework to assist practitioners in identifying the key processes in the behaviour change process. This framework then allows practitioners to build interventions around key variables to try and ensure the success of a campaign. Uutela et al. (2004) state theory must be integrated into methods and made explicit in evaluation, indicating the integration of theory into the whole campaign process.

Second, the models themselves focus on individual decision-making and therefore lack an emphasis on wider social, environmental, and cultural factors. This is an important consideration in using theoretical models, although it does not stop you taking these factors into account separately through your analysis of the target group and your needs assessment (see Chapters 3 and 4 for more detail on these areas).

Finally, there are criticisms specific to each model. The TTM is sometimes criticized for its stages. A study by Aveyard et al. (2009) that examined stage matching to improve effectiveness of behaviour change interventions suggests that the TTM was not effective in inducing stage movement in relation to smoking cessation. Other critics consider that models should incorporate additional variables to be more effective. There has been some research to suggest that additional variables could be incorporated into the TPB. Mason and White (2008) found that attitude, subjective norm, perceived behavioural control, group norm and past behaviour were all predictive of intentions to breast self-examine. In response to this, work by Fishbein and Capella (2006) included an integrative model based on the original TPB that involves some of the wider factors such as past behaviour, personalities, media exposure and demographic variables which may be useful for future health communication efforts.

CHAPTER REVIEW

This chapter identified a series of elements in the planning phase of a campaign. These include formulating SMART aims and objectives and identifying methods and channels that are linked to objectives. Recommendations centre on ensuring objectives are SMART and clearly matched to channels of communication and methods. This chapter also discussed the importance of identifying and including stakeholders in campaign design and recommends inclusion of a range of stakeholders in practice.

Then the chapter identified the importance of theoretical models in the practice of campaign planning and design. It was recommended that all campaigns that have behavioural change aims should be grounded in theoretical constructs to increase the likelihood of a successful outcome. A variety of practical ways that practitioners can incorporate theoretical models into campaigns through a series of case studies and activities were examined.

This chapter has:

- examined the formulation of aims and objectives and identified ways to link these to methods;
- analysed the role of stakeholders in health campaigns;
- explored theoretical models and their application in practice to campaign design and development.

FURTHER READING

Corcoran, N (ed.) (2007) *Communicating health strategies for health promotion*. Sage, London.
Davies, M and Macdowall, W (eds) (2006) *Health promotion theory*. Open University Press, Maidenhead.
Nutbeam, D and Harris, E (2004) *Theory in a nutshell: a guide to health promotion theory, 2nd edition*. McGraw-Hill, Maidenhead.

Starting the campaign process

This chapter will consider the starting points for undertaking a campaign. It focuses on identifying the main topic and formulating a rationale that justifies these decisions. Locations and settings for campaigns will also be examined. The issues associated with primary and secondary data collection will be outlined and different data collection methods discussed. The use of the existing evidence base and application of current interventions in practice will also be considered.

This chapter aims to:

- examine ways health topics and locations for campaigns can be identified
- identify ways to formulate a rationale for campaigns
- examine the role of primary and secondary data and evidence collection in relation to assessing need and intervention design
- consider ways to use current evidence and the application of this into practice

RATIONALES

Having selected a planning model, campaign planners need to identify what a campaign will actually do and to provide a rationale, for example, will the campaign reduce mortality or morbidity? Will it increase skills? Will it influence attitudes? Or will it change behavioural practice? To some extent these issues will have become clear through the formulation of aims and objectives and the selection of theoretical models. However, a practitioner needs to be able to justify these decisions based on evidence and research through primary and secondary data collection. This will ensure that a campaign is clearly targeted and focused and that decisions concerning the target group, location, health issue, theory, and methods are supported by evidence.

A rationale is an explanation – based on the presentation of evidence collected through a variety of means – of why the campaign has a high chance of success. The decisions that practitioners make in the planning stages of the campaign will need to be represented in this rationale. A rationale can also help to clarify the current perspectives on the health issue addressed. Tones and Green (2004: 108) suggest that 'practitioners are not always in a position to begin with a blank canvas' and a rationale can help to highlight that a campaign will need to incorporate principles or elements of existing practice. Brown et al. (2006) suggest that a health issue that is influenced by an outside agency such as national agencies may mean that a response cannot be formulated without outside support. This is also generally acknowledged at the planning stage to ensure effective working partnerships and to limit duplication of effort.

FORMULATING A RATIONALE

Every campaign requires a clear rationale explaining why the campaign is necessary. Formulating a rationale is more than a paper-based exercise, as it is recognized that decision-makers often require a rationale (McKenzie et al. 2005). Those controlling finance, for example, want to know what their money is being spent on and why a campaign should be funded. A rationale should capture why a campaign is being undertaken, who it will target, what it will do, and the main reasoning behind this. Therefore a rationale should address as a minimum the following five points:

- what the main health issue is and why;
- who the main target group is and why;
- what the main methods are that will be used and why;
- where the campaign will be centred and why;
- what the benefits or outcomes will be for the main target group.

McKenzie et al. (2005) propose a rationale triangle for developing the rationale process (see Figure 3.1).

At the top of the triangle is a statement of why the issue is important, together with supporting data. The process should then be narrowed down to the target group and the proposed health issue. A solution to the campaign should be provided as well as what can be gained from the campaign. A statement about why a campaign will be successful comes at the bottom of the triangle. All this information should be appropriately referenced using up-to-date, reliable, sources.

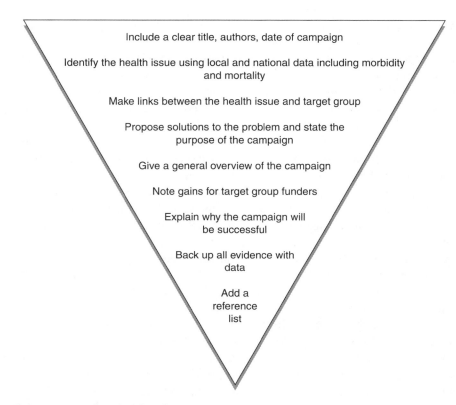

Include a clear title, authors, date of campaign

Identify the health issue using local and national data including morbidity and mortality

Make links between the health issue and target group

Propose solutions to the problem and state the purpose of the campaign

Give a general overview of the campaign

Note gains for target group funders

Explain why the campaign will be successful

Back up all evidence with data

Add a reference list

Figure 3.1   Rationale triangle
Source: Adapted from McKenzie et al. (2005).

In order to write a rationale and plan a campaign effectively, data will need to be collected from a range of sources. The health information pyramid may be helpful for research, first proposed by Annett and Rifkin (1995). In this pyramid, ten health-related aspects are identified for data collection. These include collecting research on health policy, educational services, health services, social services, physical environment, socio-economic environment, disease and disability, community composition, community and organization structure and community capacity. In addition, they suggest a three-prong method comprising: (1) key informant interviews; (2) field observations; and (3) a review of current existing documentation.

SELECTING HEALTH ISSUES

Some practitioners will already have decided specific campaign topics. This may be because they work within a service that is linked to a specific health issue.

Alternatively, funding may have been allocated for work on a health issue or with a specific target group. This makes choosing a broad category of health fairly straightforward, although which actual element of the health issue will be targeted may not be so clear. For example, in a coronary heart disease organization, should the campaign focus on reducing cholesterol levels, increasing physical activity, changing elements in diet, recognizing signs of a heart attack, or some other issue?

If no clear health issue has yet been decided, or there are a number of possible areas that could be chosen, then the health issues will need to be prioritized. Priorities may differ between different individuals and groups, in which case the planning process can help to achieve a consensus. In addition, a priority from the perspective of a stakeholder may be different from that of health practitioners, which may be different again to that of the target group. Factors such as geography, environment, personal opinions and beliefs can all influence how priorities are chosen. Generally, objective planning priorities are chosen according to prevalence, severity, mortality and morbidity. However, budgets, resources, skills, experience, stakeholders, political climate, social and cultural factors, and the ease and cost of the solution are also important.

It is possible that criteria will need to be developed to inform the decision process (see case study 3.1). Mavalankar and Abreu (2002) in their work on renovation of hospital facilities suggest developing criteria from the findings and using a scoring system to rank these into priority order. Levy et al. (2004) sort their data into 'themes' from the qualitative data collected to enable clearer discussion of key points. Therefore it is important to develop a framework that answers questions such as: Which has the highest mortality rate? Which has the highest morbidity rate? Which is the most easiest to address? Which is the cheapest to address? Which will have the most long term impact?

Activity 3.1:   Prioritizing health issues

1   You are working on a national campaign in your country to address a health issue. Rank the following five issues that could impact on health in order of what you think is the most important issue, to the least important issue (1 = high, 5 = low) in your country.

HIV prevention   access to safe drinking water   good road infrastructures no smoking policies inside workplaces   colon cancer screening

2   What made you put your priority first? Or last?
3   If you were working in a developing country or a developed country would your list change?
4   If you were going to work on one of these issues nationally, what secondary data would you try and collect to help you make an evidence-based decision on what should be a priority?

Case study 3.1: Selecting priority issues through an interactive workshop

Vallely et al. (2007) used participatory methodologies to develop community dialogue in the context of a microbicide trial feasibility study for women at risk of HIV/STIs in Tanzania and collected data through one-day community workshops. The women undertook a variety of tasks through a workshop including the following:

1 *Listing, scoring, ranking key issues*
   Lists were placed on the floor and participants placed plant seeds next to issues they rated as important (using a scale of 3 seeds = most important, to 1 seed = least important).
2 *Chapati diagramming*
   Participants drew circles to represent priority issues, the bigger the circle the higher the priority. The circles were used to promote discussion on key priority issues.
3 *Pair-wise ranking*
   This was used for participants to identify which issue was the more important of two given issues. Two issues were compared together, and then the group chose which one of the two issues was the most important. The final ranking showed that some issues were rated as more important than others and thus were higher priorities.

ANALYSING A HEALTH ISSUE

Identifying a health issue such as HIV/AIDS or cancer can be quite straightforward as the mortality and morbidity levels connected with these are widely recognized. The selection of the elements of this health issue that will form the basis of a campaign may be more complex. It is not enough to say a campaign will focus on a broad health issue. Health issues need to be broken down into the factors that influence behaviours (for example, using a condom to prevent an STI) and factors that in turn need to be targeted to change this behaviour (such as promoting positive attitudes to the purchasing and wearing of a condom). This will require more detailed knowledge of the target group and its response to elements that can impact on behaviour. Data will need to be collected, ideally using a theoretical model as the basis to identify elements that can impact on behaviour changes, for example, a campaign that has identified CHD as an issue might have chosen to focus on high cholesterol as an issue in a certain target group. The campaign might use the Health Belief Model (Becker 1974) as the basis for its campaign. It would therefore be interested in identifying elements such as benefits, barriers, susceptibility and severity in relation to high cholesterol and reducing high cholesterol. The findings from this information would then form the basis of which elements will be targeted to produce the desired outcomes. The focus for this campaign could then be to reduce high cholesterol by reducing two barriers to change and promoting two specific benefits cited as important by the target group.

Activity 3.2:   Designing questions to assist campaign focus

You are working on a campaign to reduce diabetes in a group of overweight females. Choose one theoretical model to focus your campaign on from Chapter 2.

1   What questions could you ask this group based on the theoretical model that you have chosen?
2   Would your intervention be designed differently if you had chosen a different theoretical model?

SETTINGS AND LOCATION

Planners need to consider the setting and location in which a campaign will take place. Where health information is accessed is important. There is a distinct overlap between the channels of communication and the *settings* where the target group live, work and play. This link is recognized by a number of authors as the move from people to place becomes more popular (Sivaram et al. 2007) and the emphasis has shifted away from individuals and more towards environments (Yancey et al. 2004).

Location can also be important in relation to health behaviours. Holzner and Oetomo (2004) note that wider political or structural factors influence dominant discourses in Indonesia in relation to sexual health. Indonesia characterizes youth sexuality as unhealthy and warns of the dangers of sex, rather than promoting responsibility and choice. This impacts not only on sexual health dialogue in communities, but also on the availability of condoms. Tanaka et al. (2008) state that HIV risk after displacement increases dramatically particularly in relation to transaction sexual behaviours (for example, sexual intercourse for food or money) – although location is clearly not the sole influence on health, as other factors are important.

It is also important to identify whether your target group spend time in a location where they may engage in riskier behaviours than usual. Nightclubs or pubs are a possible example of this in relation to alcohol or illegal drug use among younger people. As with the HIV example, location is not the only influencing factors: factors such as peer pressure, desire to have a 'good time' and other mitigating factors may be very important to health communication.

Research has indicated that the wider environmental variables, such as access to recreational facilities, may also impact on health promotion. Although some of this research is contradictory (see, for example, Moore et al. (2008) and Abercrombie et al. (2008) and their research on recreational facilities), there is still a possibility that access to a service or facility, especially for those who have less time, or are less inclined to participate, may be a barrier. Jilcott et al. (2007) suggest that in some inner city areas supermarkets with healthy, inexpensive foods are not available. Health campaigns in relation to healthy eating would then need to take these issues into account.

Potential settings are varied and there are several different ways in which they can be utilized to reach campaign goals. Organizational and community channels can reach priority populations through a range of means (McKenzie et al. 2005) including community activities, newsletters or bulletin boards. Campaigns can also take advantage of the setting, for example, using cinemas to advertise health messages. This has the advantage of a captive audience that may not be easily reached through other channels and could be used to both advertise and launch campaigns. Peddecord et al. (2008) used cinema advertising of silent movie theatre slides to promote the flu vaccine in English and Spanish in the USA. They propose that this may be a viable way to promote vaccine and other health issues in that this was demonstrated to be a cost-effective way to reach a diverse audience with one message. Another example comes from Minc et al. (2007) who describe a radio programme *Jailbreak*. This programme is broadcast to prisoners and the local community using a community radio station in Australia and is designed to address health issues in the prison community.

Alternatively, campaigns may make use of a whole setting approach (see case study 3.2). In reality, there is a clear overlap between health campaigns and the locations that they are related to. One of the distinct advantages of setting for health communication campaigns, as highlighted by Corcoran and Garlick (2007), is the 'normalization' of aspects of health. For example, if sexual health information was given to everyone in a workplace and discussed in a more open context, this might encourage a growing dialogue of discussion and encourage more people to access sexual health services when needed. This dialogue of discussion is important in health campaigns as this translates more mass media elements of campaigns into more intrapersonal and interpersonal communication.

Case study 3.2: Promoting sun safety at cricket matches

Lynch and Dunn (2003) examined the use of scoreboard advertising to promote the Australian SunSmart programme at one cricket ground in Australia. The rationale for using this channel was that it is a potential advertisement that can be seen by everyone. Cricket was seen as a good setting as the sport is a popular pastime and is well attended by young men. It is also played through the hottest part of the day (over lunch) and not all the seating is shaded. The message was the same as the Australian SunSmart message: 'Slip! On a shirt, Slop! On the sunscreen, Slap! On a broad brimmed hat' (2003: 489).

Advertisements appeared on the scoreboard 5–10 second intervals at scheduled breaks in play and pre/post match. They were shown approximately seven times a day. There were also SunSmart posters on display, clothing, hats and sunscreen on sale and the cricket team wore hats and glasses where practical. Recall was just over 15 per cent and those who did see this message were engaged in higher levels of sun protective behaviours. For more information, see Lynch and Dunn (2003).

Effective communication depends on a clear understanding of the target audience (Peattie 2007). Aspects include: who accesses the setting, the purpose of the setting, the behaviour of people in that setting, and the possible advantages and disadvantages of that setting. A number of key questions need to be asked when choosing a setting for campaigns. These include the following:

- Does the whole target group access this location?
- What is the main purpose of this location?
- What other healthy/unhealthy behaviours are practised in this location and will they impact on your campaign?
- What are the potential channels for campaign messages in this location?
- Are there any pitfalls or challenges in using this location and how will you overcome these?

Activity 3.3:   Choosing a setting for road safety messages

1 Choose one setting that could be used to promote a 'designated driver' campaign. (This refers to a situation where one person does not drink alcohol and remains the vehicle driver all evening.)
2 Once you have chosen the setting, ask yourself the five key questions listed above.
3 Would you still use this setting based on your answers to these questions?

Case study 3.3:   Feasibility of using wine shops in India for HIV Prevention

Sivaram et al. (2007) examined the possibility of using wine shops in India for the prevention of HIV. Wine shops are community-based licensed locations for alcohol consumption both on premises or to take away. Wine shops are seen as potentially useful for three main reasons: there are high rates of hazardous alcohol drinking in India; wine shops samples have higher rates of sexual risk behaviours: and alcohol is associated with higher risk sexual behaviours.

The study indicates there is potential for HIV prevention in wine shops for a number of reasons. These include the fact that they are a close private space, patrons are regular customers and are familiar with each other, and the shop offers a space where topics such as sexual health are not taboo. There are also several possible locations for condom machines and wine staff are receptive to the campaign and amenable. One disadvantage, however, may be that alcohol may impact on the ability to foster safe sexual behaviours.

See Sivaram et al. (2007) for more information.

Problems of settings and locations

Settings and locations can sometimes hinder health communication and information exchanges. This may in part be because people cannot access those settings or because the setting itself may not be conducive to that message. For example, a long and detailed message on a billboard would not be read by passing drivers as they would not have time to read the information. Some settings may not be conducive to the specified behaviour, for example, a setting that has alcohol may skew judgements, or peer pressure may mean messages are not adhered to. Placement of messages in the wrong place may also mean people do not see the message. Other policies and practices may not be conducive to change. A study by Hemmick and McCarthy (2007) notes that despite efforts to promote emergency contraception pills accessibility in colleges and universities in one US state, concerns about controversy, and prohibition by university policies prevented provision.

Other problems stem from the resistance of a group to interventions (Tones and Green 2004). This is problematic throughout the communication process and only clear *formative evaluation* and planning can ensure this effect is lessened (see Chapter 7 for more on formative evaluation). In health promotion efforts, Whitelaw et al. (2001) suggest a 'bottom-up' approach to settings, rather than a top-down one, might be more effective. The practical implication of this for campaign design is the need to involve the target audience from the intended setting in the campaign planning and pre-testing of materials.

$\gg$

Activity 3.4: HPV (Human papillomavirus) vaccine promotion in a community setting

A study in Malaysia by Wong (2009) notes that public ignorance, confusion about the vaccine and infection, socio-economic cultural sensitivities about an STI vaccine and vaccine cost all impact on efforts to promote the HPV vaccine in Malaysia. Malaysian communities have strong traditional values and higher socio-economic power lies with men who are generally more economically active than women and play an important part in decision-making. Efforts to promote the vaccine raise a number of concerns. These include the idea that, by providing vaccines against STIs, teenage sexual behaviour is being condoned. In addition, any solutions need to consider that a large proportion of the population are Muslim and interventions need to consider cultural and religious sensitivities.

1 What would you do in a community setting to promote the prevention of HPV infection through vaccination?
2 Who would you involve in message design?
3 What settings might be appropriate for a campaign to promote this vaccine?
4 Create one message based on the information above that is tailored to your chosen setting.

DATA COLLECTION

All campaigns will need at some point to collect data. This might be for the rationale phases as described earlier, it might be to help identify a health issue, location or target group, or it might be for the evaluation process (see Chapter 7). However data is used, the processes for collecting data remain very similar. In some instances a 'needs assessment' might be undertaken which incorporates a range of these elements (the health issue, location, target group, and so on) into one assessment. Any data collection process will go through similar steps which include identifying the resources and ways to collect data, collecting the data and analyzing the data. If practitioners want to complete a whole needs assessment to help them identify issues such as locations or target groups, they may wish to undertake additional steps. McKenzie et al. (2005) suggest the six steps in assessing need in health promotion which can be applied to campaigns design: identifying methods to locate data; collecting the data; analysing the data; identifying the health problem; identifying the health focus; and validating findings.

The next part of this chapter will consider ways to collect primary and secondary data alongside issues associated with data collection, validity and reliability of these processes.

Collecting primary data

Both quantitative and qualitative methods have an important role in campaign planning. What kind of information a specific campaign needs will depend on the participants and the context (Farquhar et al. 2006). Farquhar et al. propose a number of qualitative methods to enable data collection at each stage of the planning process. For example, when the campaign is in the initial stage of problem analysis, reviews of documents, in-depth interviews with the community or organizations or group interviews with the steering committee may be helpful. There are a number of ways primary data can help to plan campaigns. These can be single methods such as focus groups, interviews, questionnaires, surveys, field observations, visual or oral techniques, or a combination of these. In addition, a rapid appraisal could also be undertaken.

Rapid appraisal (RA)

One method used in health promotion and public health work that can prove useful in campaign planning is rapid appraisal (RA). This is a technique that allows collection of data in a community through participatory research methods. Projects may range from relatively small-scale to complex large-scale projects.

Research suggests that RA is more commonly used in developing countries, probably because of its strong emphasis on community participation (Pepall et al. 2006). Other advantages include the low cost and the fact they can often be conducted over a short period of time. See case study 3.4 for an example of this. Thus, RA can be used in a variety of ways that help with planning or allocating resources, as well as identifying key health or social issues.

Pepall et al. suggest there are some limitations to using the rapid appraisal techniques. Interview respondents may take a one-sided view of the community and therefore bias the results. In addition, reliance solely on secondary data will also not give you an accurate reflection of the whole community. Reliance on single sources of information (for example, just interviews) is not recommended.

Case study 3.4:   Rapid participatory assessment by a radio station

Pepall et al. (2006) undertook a rapid participatory assessment (RPA) examining health and social needs assessment with the view to developing a communication strategy for a radio station (Heart line Bali FM) in a small village in Indonesia.

There were two main phases to data collection, although there was also some pre-planning work in relation to identifying interviewees prior to the data collection stage. The first phase took two weeks and included communication with stakeholders, collection of information in relation to the community needs and examination of community assets. The second phase lasted one week, and included the key methods of rapid appraisal strategies. Some 60–90 minute interviews with key informants (guided by semi-structured questionnaires), informal discussions and field observations (for example physical features of community) all took place.

Focus groups

An essential aspect of a focus group is the interaction between the data collectors and the participants (Mitchell and Branigan 2000). Focus groups and open-ended interviews offer the advantage of obtaining information on individual and community perceptions on specific topics and enabling extensive exploration of topics (Levy et al. 2008). Focus groups can also allow trust-building relationships between different groups who may subsequently all be involved in the latter stages of a campaign (Cristancho et al. 2008).

A discussion in a focus group is not simply a general conversation: it is a focused discussion on a topic, such as the design of a leaflet or access to a service. The data this produces can then be used to inform campaign design, delivery, and implementation. There are different guidelines suggested for focus groups, depending on the audience. Kraak and Pelletier (1998) note that focus groups with children who do not know each other work better as it helps to avoid peer-led influences. They also suggest familiar surroundings, splitting boys and girls, and the use of a younger trained peer are important. Other research on focus groups has suggested more interactive styles of focus groups might be useful. See case studies 3.5 and 3.6.

Case study 3.5:   Adapted focus groups

Cristancho et al. (2008) undertook a community-based participatory assessment of the barriers to health care access and use among rural Hispanic immigrants. They used a modified approach to data collection which consisted of focus groups and small group discussion combined, which they term 'focused small group discussion'. These discussions took place after a community event or activity and did not involve any formal recruitment strategies. No usual means of transcription or recording, such as audio-tapes, were used.

The study suggests that language and cultural barriers can interfere with efforts to access health care. Thus the groups were conducted in Spanish, and promotional flyers were also written in Spanish and distributed through locations such as Mexican grocery stores, churches, public libraries, and by community leaders.

Interviews, questionnaires and surveys

Interviews are usually conducted one-to-one via face-to-face interventions or telephone, though they may also be done via email and in small groups. The format of the interview depends on what kind of information is needed, but often interviews follow a structure (or are semi-structured) based on the issues needing to be discussed.

Questionnaires and surveys have the advantage of being able to ask a variety of types of question. One common way of collecting data is a written questionnaire. This method has the advantage of reaching a wide audience in a short period of time, even covering a large geographical area, and it can be low in cost (McKenzie et al. 2005).

There are a number of techniques that can help increase response rates, and ensure a good design of a questionnaire. Saks and Allsop (2008) suggest, for example, that all interviewers should be trained, and that this training should be standardized. Questionnaires should be written with a cover letter and pre-paid envelope (if posting). Follow-up then needs to be arranged. Questionnaires must all be well designed and specifically linked to the questions that require answers, rather than for collecting general information that will not be used again. It is also worth noting that analysis of data from interviews in particular can be time-consuming to analyse correctly.

Field observations

Field observation is sometimes neglected in health communication research, yet can have a number of uses. It can ensure that what is being reported is actually taking place. Observations included in an evaluation of physical activity interventions, for example, have been used to ensure that the outdoor exercise rates are similar to those reported (Kerr et al. 2001; Reger et al. 2002). In addition, it can give you a 'feel' for the community and what is going on, what resources are available and what the area is like in general. Pepall et al. (2006) in their examination of health and social needs used field observations as part of their rapid appraisal to note physical features of the area, as well as factors such as relationship features (interactions between older and younger people). This method therefore can take into account anything that might have an impact on the main health issues being examined such as resources, facilities, housing conditions, safe places to exercise or play, and so on, alongside being used in evaluation purposes.

Other visual and oral methods

There are ways to collect data that do not rely on traditional techniques. Bust et al. (2008) suggest the use of photo-elicitation. This consists of giving the target group pictures such as those that could be used in a campaign and seeking feedback to assist campaign design. Other visual and oral methods might be helpful where literacy levels are low. Methods include art forms, such as dance, drama, song, storytelling, or drawing. Visual methods might be particularly useful when dealing with children. Kortesluoma et al. (2008) looked at how children expressed pain through drawings, Pearce et al. (2009) gave children cameras to photograph physical activity and food influences, and Piko and Bak (2006) examined 5–11-year-olds' lay beliefs on health, illness, and health promotion through drawing and writing.

Case study 3.6: Focus groups for the design of cancer-screening materials

Wiehagen et al. (2007) used 'projective techniques' to undertake focus groups in the design of colorectal cancer-screening materials. Participants were split into design teams and given a range of art and craft supplies to help them design visual layouts for materials. They found that males chose blue more frequently and females chose warm, bright colours. They also found participants made liberal use of colour and chose a selection of images that they thought related to information about colon cancer. Participants expressed different opinions in relation to the content of materials. Although the authors suggest caution in the use of this technique at the moment, this does suggest that focus groups can be turned into engaging and lively experiences.

Issues in primary data collection

There are a number of issues concerning the collection of primary data. These include the more obvious challenges such as time, resources, and skills. Focus groups can be time-consuming and expensive and they require expertise to run (Mitchell and Branigan 2000). There are similar disadvantages with interviews – indeed, they are usually even more time-consuming. Interviews do not always obtain accurate or honest answers to your questions. In addition, cultural and behavioural factors may mean some people are reluctant to share information – especially on taboo or sensitive subjects with those collecting data. Bosmans et al. (2006) found when using focus groups with adolescents and adults to discuss sexual and reproductive health programmes in the Democratic Republic of Congo that, on the whole, adults felt uncomfortable talking about sex and sexuality, for example, they never used the words 'sex' or 'sexuality' in focus group dialogue.

Questionnaires may also have a low response rate. The response rate varies depending on distribution and return techniques. Incentives and pre-paid return envelopes may increase response rates. Saks and Allsop (2008) state that postal questionnaires are poor in avoiding a response bias, and may not produce high quality answers although they do report telephone questionnaires may achieve a higher response rate.

Reinert et al. (2008) suggest several lessons to follow in data collection. These are based on a study of data collection in faith-based organizations. They include pilot testing, using back-up plans, and safeguarding data. Before any data is collected, ethical approval should be obtained from the local provider. In the case of primary data collection, you will need to obtain consent from participants and provide clear information about the purpose of the data collection and what the data will be used for.

Collecting secondary data

There are a number of potential sources of secondary data. These will provide the evidence base for health-related practice. Corcoran and Garlick suggest that 'for health promotion to be successful there is a need to look at evidence critically and apply what works in order to demonstrate effectiveness' (2007: 140). Corcoran and Garlick refer to a number of sources of evidence in health practice. They include electronic bibliographic databases, electronic or paper journals, government or other organization documentation, and grey literature. Whatever secondary data is used, it will need to be appraised critically. How data is collected and used will depend on a number of issues such as location, health issue, and the availability of the data.

Specific locations in a community can also provide data specifically for the health issues you are focusing on. Accident and emergency departments, local councils, local health promotion departments, NGOs working in the area, universities, and local supermarkets can all be rich sources of information. There are a number of questions that you will need to ask when you have secondary data as it won't all fit your purpose. Questions include:

- Does the material have any bias?
- Has the material been published by a reputable source?
- Are the results reliable and valid?
- Is there any missing data?
- Is the publication recent?
- Are the methods of collecting the data clearly explained?
- Is the sample used in data collection representative of the population?
- Does the evidence agree with or contradict other findings?
- Can the evidence/results be translated into practice?

Note that even if there is a bias, or the data is old, this does not necessarily mean that it cannot be used – merely that caution must be exercised in interpreting the results.

Activity 3.5: Source validity and reliability

Choose a health issue that you are interested in and identify one source of information that you could use if you were designing a campaign in that area.

1 Using the questions listed for checking data above, ask yourself the list of questions in relation to the source that you have.
2 Do you think your source is an appropriate and useful source of information for your campaign based on your answers to these questions?

Validity and reliability

As with any data collection technique, there are questions of reliability and validity. Some problems concern bias. Tones and Green (2004) note that results from rapid appraisals can be biased if other options are not sought, especially if the community uses information from only one perspective. They suggest rapid appraisal techniques work best when following an agenda established by the community.

Triangulation of methods is important to ensure reliability and validity of findings. This can help to prevent a one-sided view, and reduce errors and prejudice coming from one source (Pepall et al. 2006). Triangulation is the process by which data from one source is validated (or in some cases rejected) when compared with data from at least two other sources or data collection methods (Brown et al. 2006). When collecting data, therefore, it is important to use a range of methods and sources to ensure that the data collected is valid and reliable.

Several biases may exist that may affect campaign outcomes. They include response bias to needs assessments that take place. Typically, people are busy with their everyday lives (Potvin et al. 2003), therefore, setting aside time to be involved in a campaign may be problematic. This may mean that those involved in needs assessments are not the actual people whose views you are seeking. Pepall et al. (2006) suggest that the use of interpreters may also bias findings in relation to inaccurate translation of information. The spoken views relayed by translators may be altered slightly in the process and so meanings can be missed.

Chinn et al. (2006) note that factors associated with non-participation in a physical activity promotion trial included being male, being a smoker, living in a more deprived areas, and rating their health as poorer. They also attached less importance to physical activity for the maintenance of health. This illustrates that there is a possibility that those who are engaged in a data collection process may not always be the ones who are being targeted, and also that a data collection process may serve to increase inequalities rather than reduce them.

Activity 3.6:   Including the excluded

1   How might you go about including those people who might be excluded from a traditional needs assessment?
2   Based on what you have read in this chapter so far, what methods might you use?

An additional problem is the bias of practitioners themselves. It can be difficult to be objective about data, especially if it is an area that interests you. Stepping back and relinquishing the role of 'expert' can be difficult. In addition, practitioners themselves may bias responses to data collection in their questions or their manner. This is another reason why data should always be collected from more than one source with a mix of primary and secondary data to try and minimize any disparities.

Case study 3.7:   Stop stroke pre-campaign phases

Redfern et al. (2008) developed an intervention to improve risk factor management after stroke. Their pre-campaign phases (which they call pre-clinical theoretical phase) consisted of the following steps:

1   A systematic review of risk factor management to evaluate effectiveness of interventions. They conducted searches through electronic databases, using recognized key words, and electronic searches of individual journals, databases and policy documents.
2   A statistical analysis of the management of secondary prevention in a sample group using the South London stroke register.
3   A series of exploratory qualitative interviews of patient experiences of secondary prevention using patients from the stroke register.
4   A professional observation study to investigate how prevention advice is given and received through two non-participation observations in a health setting.
5   A content analysis of patient information literature from local health services and patient organizations.

Data was then collated into key findings and each was addressed in turn in relation to proposed solutions. This then allowed the formulation of key aims of the campaign.

AWARENESS OF CURRENT CAMPAIGNS AND THE USE OF EXISTING CAMPAIGNS

It is important to be aware of what resources already exist. New campaigns do not always require new resources, for example, a target group could ask for a range of health leaflets in a different language. Research indicated that they already exist, so the question might be whether a new set of leaflets should be made or existing leaflets moved to a better location. It may be that a whole new campaign does not need to be undertaken and that an adaptation to an existing campaign is possible. For a more detailed discussion of applicability and transferability, see Wang et al. (2005) and Corcoran and Garlick (2007).

Brunton et al. (2007) suggest that, when looking for evidence to inform the design of health promotion studies, questions arise concerning: (1) effectiveness; (2) feasibility; and (3) acceptability. First, is this intervention going to work in the proposed setting? Second, will it be do-able in the proposed setting? And, finally, will the intervention be accepted by the proposed target group? Secondary data that is used to provide a rationale for campaign planning will need to consider these questions in some detail as the more evidence that can be accumulated that interventions work in specific groups or areas, the stronger the rationale. Likewise, any problems experienced in studies also need to be considered to eliminate these from the planned campaign.

CHAPTER REVIEW

This chapter has considered the role of rationales and of undertaking an assessment of campaign needs to justify campaign planning decisions. Ways to identify health issues and locations and settings for campaigns are discussed and it is recommended that careful consideration of locations is needed for campaign interventions. This chapter has examined ways to undertake data collection processes through primary and secondary data collection and the issues associated with using these methods. This chapter recommends that both primary and secondary data collection should be undertaken to ensure that campaign planning is robust and evidence-based. Validity and reliability of evidence are also considered in the context of campaigns.

This chapter has:

- examined the construction of a rationale to ensure interventions are appropriately evidence-based;
- analysed ways to identify specific health issues, locations and settings for campaigns;
- identified a range of primary and secondary data collection methods that can be utilized in the campaign planning process.

FURTHER READING

Coles, L and Porter, E (2009) *Public health skills*. Blackwell Publishing, London.

Douglas, J, Lloyd, C and Sidell, M (2007) Using research to plan multidisciplinary public health interventions pp. 297–326 in Earle, S, Lloyd, C E, Sidell, M and Spurr, S (eds) *Theory and practice in promoting public health*. Sage, London.

A number of textbooks that examine qualitative research methods will help with primary data collection sources. Two recent ones that might be of interest are:

Berg, B L (2007) *Qualitative research methods for the social sciences, 6th edition*. Pearson, London.

Saks, M and Allsop, J (2008) *Researching health*. Sage, London.

Target groups

This chapter will examine the social and psychological factors that characterize target groups. It includes an examination of social factors such as age, sex, ethnicity, religion and culture. Psychological factors that will be explored include attitudes, beliefs and values. Defining a target group and tailoring information to target groups will also be considered.

This chapter aims to:

- identify the impact of social, structural and psychological factors to health communication programmes
- analyze the relationship between social, structural and psychological factors in campaigns
- explore ways to map a target group and their characteristics through theoretical and practical examples

CHARACTERISTICS OF TARGET GROUPS

There is a complex relationship between social, structural, and psychological factors. In relation to campaigns, this means that some factors that characterize a target group might not be as simple as they first seem. Identifying a target group based on simple factors such as age or sex may be reasonably straightforward, but actually what influences the health status and behaviour of a target group is much more complex than this. Social variables such as age, sex, ethnicity, religion and spiritual beliefs interlink with structural factors such as location, occupation, housing and environment. These in turn are linked to psychological variables such as knowledge, attitudes, beliefs and values.

Identifying the whole spectrum of influences on health is difficult. For example, age might predict education levels, or housing location. Sex might predict beliefs and knowledge levels. Religion might impact on self-esteem or attitudes. However, it might not be age or sex that predicts how a target group behave or what they believe but other variables such as education, country of residence, or current occupation. White and Cash (2004) note that there are differences in male and female health status across age groups geographically. A 20-year-old female does not have the same health status as every other 20-year-old in the country. In addition, characteristics of a target group such as sex and religion combine with additional factors such as 'content of the message, timing, social context, community norms … [and] … cultural attitudes' (Tanvatanakul et al. 2007: 174).

Adequate consideration of target group characteristics is certainly not universal in current campaigns. Research suggests that gender-specific and culturally relevant health promotion interventions are needed, as many interventions do not take these characteristics into consideration (Courtenay et al. 2002). It can be hypothesized that if practitioners do not take into account characteristics of target groups, a vital key to changing attitude or behaviour could be missed.

SOCIAL VARIABLES

Age

Age impacts on a number of factors in relation to health. First, it can influence health behaviours and health risk and, second, it influences the sources accessed for health information. In relation to health behaviours, simple factors such as legality (for example, being over 16, 18 or 21) can have an impact on health behaviours. Alternatively, health issues may be more prevalent in certain age groups (such as osteoporosis being more common in older people, or cot death linked to young babies).

Take the example of alcohol. In Australia, alcohol use peaks with early adulthood and declines with age. This means that younger people have more problematic alcohol-related behaviour than older people (Livingston and Room 2009). A similar pattern can be observed in the UK and some other European countries. However, in China alcohol use increases with age (especially in rural areas) (Mao and Wu 2007). Thus an alcohol prevention campaign in China would probably focus on different age ranges than an alcohol prevention campaign in Australia.

Research suggests that different age groups use different sources of health information. Cotton and Gupta (2004) suggest that age (along with income and education) is a predictor of using online or offline health information, with those who are younger being more likely to access health information online. The internet has also been suggested by Tanvatanakul et al. (2007) as a source more frequently used by younger age groups. Television, radio and newspapers were more frequently used by older age groups. Närhi and Helakorpi (2007) indicate that in relation to medical information, older people consider doctors to be their most common source of medical information but younger age groups were found to prefer sources that do not involve a health professional such as the internet. This indicates that information preference could be different based on age. In campaigns this is clearly important as any channel of communication used must be one that the target group are comfortable with and likely to access.

Activity 4.1:   Health information sources based on age

Identify in your local area what the main sources of health information might be for the following groups:

1   Adults over 70.
2   Children under 11.
3   Older teenagers (16–19).

There may be inconsistencies in what a target group considers as an appropriate channel of communication. For example, in secondary schools, male and female children (5–12th grade) indicated that their mother was the primary source for childhood healthcare information. There was some difference between ages, however, and the younger of the groups were more likely to approach their mother first but older children approach their friends first (Ackard and Neumark-Sztainer 2001). This may indicate that the importance of the mother as an information source may decrease with increasing age, or illustrate that older age groups are able to access more sources of information. Research in Japan (Nonoyama et al. 2007) found that it was uncommon for adolescents to go to their parents first for sexual health information. Adolescents in Japan used friends, magazines and the television as sources of information as it is uncommon for adolescents to approach parents, and rare for adolescents to access an environment where they can talk openly about sex. These two studies suggest therefore that other variables such as culture, health topic and accessibility to information may impact on communication channels. It is therefore important to check which channels of communication are the best ones for the facilitation of health messages.

Sex and gender

Like age, there are numerous ways in which sex and gender can influence health. There are different definitions of the terms sex and gender. For the purposes of this book, 'sex' refers to being either male or female; 'gender' refers to the masculine and feminine characteristics that either sex may display. Sex differences in health status exist in mortality and morbidity rates across a range of health areas. There are a number of reasons for this and some of these are important in relation to campaigns. First, men may engage in riskier behaviours, have riskier beliefs and report poorer medical compliance and preventive behaviours (for example, self-examinations) than women (Courtenay et al. 2002). Other differences in health behaviour are linked to healthy lifestyle behaviours. For example, female adolescents typically have more sexual health knowledge than males, and males have more liberal attitudes than females towards sexual health (Coleman and Testa 2007). Thus, knowledge and attitudes held by males and females may impact directly on health behaviour. In addition, social roles are important in health campaigns. Kerr-Corrêa et al. (2007) report that for women marriage, employment and children decrease alcohol consumption, whereas divorce, unemployment and the absence of children encourage alcohol drinking. Kerr-Corrêa et al. also note that men and women have different reasons for drinking alcohol, for example, men drink alcohol to demonstrate masculinity, socially as a way to escape social control and to improve male bonding. This finding serves to illustrate one of the reasons alcohol promotion advertisements often show groups of males together enjoying each other's company away from women. It is possible that alcohol advertisements that aim to reduce drinking levels will need to illustrate male bonding in an alternative way, or challenge the ideals that alcohol is an attractive, masculine, pursuit.

Närhi and Helakorpi (2007) suggest that women are more active than men in seeking medical information and that they utilize a wider range of sources of information. This is emphasized by findings of Ackard and Neumark-Sztainer (2001) who indicate in a study of school children that boys were more likely than girls to report that they did not know where to access health information. This is important for campaigns as it suggests that the location of health information may be an important issue when focusing on campaigns aimed at males and that additional sign-posting of materials may be necessary.

Activity 4.2:   Campaigns for men and women

Ferrand et al. (2008) note that there are gender differences in relation to motivation to participate in physical activity (in a type 2 diabetes programme). Females emphasize more emotional support and pleasure from attending a group environment. Males emphasize knowledge acquisition and skills for disease control.

1   You are designing a physical activity campaign aimed at patients with type 2 diabetes from a number of GP practices. You want to aim your campaign at both men and women. What sort of messages might you include in your resources for both men and women based on the Ferrand et al. (2008) study findings?
2   Do you think you would need to create two separate campaigns? Why/why not?

In relation to campaigns, there is little research to suggest that men and women look for different information formats. Flynn et al. (2007) noted that age was a bigger predictor factor than sex in the appeal of health messages. There is, however, some evidence to suggest that there could be differences in information sources by sex. Bessinger et al. (2004) suggest that radio messages appealed more to women in an STI media campaign. In addition, gender stereotyping may prevent some forms of communication (Nonoyama et al. 2007), and it is important to be aware of this. Research by Rios-Ellis et al. (2008) suggests that, in Latino culture in the USA, cultural expectations of male dominance and protection influence family and sexual relationships. Effective campaign messages will need to take these conventions into account.

Literacy levels may also inhibit the reading of some materials, or conventions may not allow women to access certain public places where health materials are available. There is a distinct difference worldwide in male over female literacy levels with nearly all least developed countries demonstrating substantial gaps between male and female literacy (UNESCO 2001). Mapping your target group clearly (see later in this chapter) will ensure that you cover these differences if they do exist.

Ethnicity

There are numerous ways in which ethnicity may impact on health. Ethnicity can be difficult to separate from culture (considered in the next section of this chapter) as most ethnic groups identify with a culture, which may be more influential on health than ethnicity. The individual effects of each are difficult to separate.

Activity 4.3: Variables that influence diet

You are working on a campaign to increase fruit and vegetable consumption in your local population.

1 What different patterns of fruit and vegetable consumption are there within different ethnic groups in your local area?
2 What factors influence the different fruit and vegetable consumption within these ethnic groups?
3 What different elements could you incorporate into messages that aim to promote fruit and vegetable consumption in these ethnic groups?

The example of sexual health and sexual behaviours demonstrates the complexity of the influence of ethnicity. Coleman and Testa (2007) in a school-based study indicate that, in the UK, there are differences between ethnic groups in sexual health knowledge, attitudes, and behaviours. For example, the lowest sexual health knowledge was found in Pakistani males, females and black African males. The highest levels of knowledge were white British males and females. White British males also have the most liberal attitudes to sexual health. Black males and females were more likely to have had sexual intercourse without contraception, more so in Black African females than Black Caribbeans. These findings illustrate the complexities surrounding ethnicity in relation to sexual health and the different sexual health needs of ethnic groups.

In most countries, research has tended to find that minority populations have poorer health outcomes than the majority population. The Office of Minority Health (2007) in the USA notes disproportionate rates of morbidity and mortality in minority ethnic groups compared to white groups. Raine et al. (2003) found Latino women (compared to African American, Asian, White and other) were less likely than other groups to use any contraception, thus putting themselves at higher risk of unplanned pregnancy and STIs.

This may not be the case with all health behaviours, however, and in some cases ethnicity may have a positive influence. Courtenay et al. (2002) notes that, although European Americans had better diet and eating practices compared to African Americans or Hispanics, they were more likely than either group to use alcohol frequently and to be a current cigarette smoker. Additional research reports that ethnicity may also have protective effects on health. Kornblau et al. (2007) note ethnic differences in body esteem that show African-American women have more favourable body esteem than whites. Possibly this is linked to different cultural norms, more positive body images, and different expectations of what is attractive.

Ethnicity can also impact on the processes of communication. Although there is little evidence to suggest how this translates into campaigns, Siminoff et al. (2006) note in cancer care communication that racial differences in the communication exchange between patient and provider illustrate that providers communicate differently with different ethnic groups. It can probably be hypothesized that this might also be the case in other forms of health communication and may be a future area of research in campaign design and development.

Culture

Culture is a dynamic process involving different beliefs and practices (Willging et al. 2006). Kreuter et al. (2003) suggest there are a number of factors that contribute to the notion of culture. These include communication patterns, individualism or collectivism, and characteristics that may not be inherently cultural but that may define culture for a group. Best et al. (2008) note that different ethnic groups express themselves in different ways based on cultural knowledge and convention. Culture is complex, for example, all white Europeans do not share a single *monolithic* culture, country, religion, education or occupation. In campaigns it is important to be able to describe the cultures and sub-cultures and consider how these relate to aspects that influence health (Kreuter et al. 2003). Work by Dodds (2002) suggests situating health topics in appropriate contexts, and using the group's own terminology.

An additional variable may be the degree of pervasion of Western medical beliefs in campaigns, especially those that aim to prevent ill-health through screening. For example, Chinese-Australian women thought western medical practitioners often lacked cultural sensitivity. They also thought the power of Western medicine was exaggerated and were less willing to accept screening because of this (Kwok and Sullivan 2007). Any efforts to encourage screening in these groups would need to address these issues.

The processes of *acculturation* can also have an impact on health. Kerr-Corrêa et al. (2007) suggest that alcohol drinking patterns and practices are changed through acculturation, for example, some Arabic groups who drink alcohol despite religious practices that deem this behaviour undesirable. This may also be the case with other health behaviours. Other research suggests clear integration of the target group with materials to ensure success. Research by Willging et al. (2006) found that the cultural concepts they included in their work with American-Indian cultures did not mesh with the realities of day-to-day life.

Kreuter et al. (2003) suggest that, when planning an intervention with a strong cultural element in it (for example, a non-English-speaking ethnic minority group), practitioners usually select an intervention from one of five categories (Table 4.1).

Table 4.1   Categories for planning culturally specific campaigns using Kreuter et al.'s (2003) five categories

Strategy	Description	Example in practice
Peripheral	Adapting or designing materials to appear culturally appropriate such as using images, colours that appeal	Adapting existing materials for Black Caribbean males by using photographs specifically related to this group
Evidential	Presenting evidence of the impact of a health issue on a specific group such as data centred on susceptibility or vulnerability	Presenting facts in a leaflet aimed at Black African women with statistics such as 'African women are more likely to be diagnosed with …'
Linguistic	Provision of materials in others of the target group such as translating existing materials	Translating a leaflet for different Asian language groups such as Urdu or Punjabi
Constituent involving	Drawing on experience of the target group and involving them in the communication process	Using Chinese women to create messages in a healthy heart leaflet and involving them in the design and distribution of this leaflet
Socio-cultural	Consider health issues in wider social contexts and include cultural aspects of the audience such as recognition of beliefs, values, and behaviours	In sexual health materials targeted at Muslim women discussion of sexual health issues is located in the context of marital relationships

The categories are peripheral, evidential, linguistic, constituent-involving and socio-cultural:

- a peripheral strategy is one that is adapted for the target group, for example, using certain images or colours that appeal to the audience;
- an evidential strategy is the presentation of evidence and its impact on that group centred around that group's vulnerability or susceptibility;
- a linguistic strategy is the provision of materials in different languages;
- a constituent-involving strategy involves using the target groups' own experience and involving them in the communication process;
- a socio-cultural strategy is one that considers health issues in a wider social context, for example, the recognition that values and beliefs impact on health behaviours.

It is suggested that a mixture of these strategies or those that include more integration with the target group are likely to result in a more effective campaign.

Activity 4.4: Five cultural strategies

Read again the description of Kreuter et al.'s (2003) five cultural strategies:

1 What are the main advantages and disadvantages of using these strategies?
2 If you were designing an intervention and you wanted to use just one of these strategies, which would you choose and why?
3 Would your decision change if you had limited money or resources? Or limited access to the target group you want to reach?

Case study 4.1:   Cultural tailoring of materials

Kreuter et al. (2003) examined cultural tailoring to a subset of a group of African American women. The project aimed to increase mammography and fruit and vegetable consumption by tailoring health messages in a magazine to cultural characteristics. To tailor information, they did the following:

1 Identified demography; age, sex, ethnicity.
2 Identified geographical area; living in one area, seeking healthcare at one of ten clinics.
3 Chose four potentially important cultural characteristics of the group; religion, collectivism, racial pride, perception of time (for example, thinking of short- or long-term health outcomes). These were selected as they were seen to be measurable, significantly different to allow tailoring and demonstrated to be associated with health beliefs and practices.

Religion and spiritual beliefs

Religion may play an important part in health. There may be differences in health in relation to different religious denominations and how religion is practised. For example, religion has been found to be protective in some health areas, such as adolescent risk behaviours (Nonnemaker et al. 2003). Religious involvement has also been associated with low alcohol consumption (Kerr-Corrêa et al. 2007). Manlove et al. (2006) suggest that parents' religious attendance and family religious activities are related to later timing of sexual initiation although religious beliefs and denomination are not. Nonnemaker et al. (2003) found both public and private religiosity ('public' meaning attendance at services and participation in religious groups and 'private' meaning frequency of prayer and importance of religion) are protective for a number of health factors, and there are some small differences between the two. Generally, however, this study found that religiosity may be protective against cigarettes, alcohol, marijuana and lower probability of ever having sexual intercourse and engaging in violence.

Religion may also facilitate health promotion behaviours. Shuval et al. (2008) found that religion was considered a facilitating factor for physical activity because of support in scriptures. The use of places of worship for a health promotion setting has also been investigated (Corcoran and Bone 2007).

Activity 4.5: Targeting physical activity to religion

You are designing a healthy heart awareness campaign aimed at reducing rates of coronary heart disease (CHD) for a group that are frequent attendees at a place of worship in your local area.

1   How could you target your messages to make them relevant to the target group by incorporating religion and religious practices into messages?

There is some research to suggest religion may be associated with poorer health behaviours. Research by Raine et al. (2003) suggests that being raised with a religion may be an indicator of non-contraceptive use, possibly because of less willingness or ability to acknowledge sexual behaviours due to prohibitions or expected social norms of that religious community. In addition, the conformity and strict moral and religious dogma associated with some religions may have negative impacts on health, such as guilt or anxiety and therefore mental health, particularly for those who do not conform to these religious ideas and values (for more on this topic, see Lucas and Lloyd 2005).

There is very little research, in relation to communication, on the role of alternative spiritual beliefs on health behaviours. This includes other life philosophies (for example, being an environmentalist with pacifist beliefs). There are also other spiritual belief philosophies, such as kabala or scientology, that may impact on health. In this instance identifying influences on the target group in relation to their beliefs is important in relation to campaigns (see section on beliefs), as these are not well documented in current research. See Activity 4.6 for an example of spiritual and cultural beliefs in campaigns.

Activity 4.6: Tailoring to philosophies

You are designing an intervention to increase physical activity levels in a group with a strong environmental and sustainable living ethos.

1   What sort of messages could be targeted to this group based on this?

Case study 4.2: Culturally targeted cancer information

A study by Kulukulualani et al. (2008) developed culturally targeted cancer education brochures specifically tailored to native Hawaiians. This study notes that native

> Hawaiians have a world-view that is influenced by 'salient cultural concepts'. This includes the land, extended family, co-operation, helpfulness and humility. Family associations are important, and the group takes precedence over individuals. Emphasis is also placed on caring for each other.
>
> The target group wanted speakers in the materials to look Hawaiian and healthy and information to incorporate Hawaiian values. This included notions of family, being part of a group, and the natural environment. Pictures illustrated Hawaiians in outdoor settings such as fishing, and friends and family caring for each other alongside incorporating common Hawaiian words and phrases into the materials.

Additional variables

There are a number of additional structural and social variables that may turn out to be more influential than the common ones previously discussed. Language, medium and location of health communication information can vary depending on social class, education (Corcoran and Corcoran 2007) and occupation. Povlsen et al. (2005) note that having little education background may mean remembering facts or new information is difficult. Occupation may also be influential in undertaking healthy or unhealthy behaviours. Jans et al. (2007) note that some occupations are more sedentary than others and other research notes that mortality rates linked to alcohol are higher among workers in the drinks industry, catering, entertainment, hospitality and some skilled trades (Baker 2008).

Other variables need to be considered depending on the characteristics of the audience. Marketing and advertising agencies group people with similar characteristics into sub-sections. These are usually categories made for groups of people who have a number of factors in common such as habits, purchasing patterns, hobbies and interests. CBS Outdoor (2009b) note their audiences to be: urbanites, shoppers (main shopper, top up shopper and retail shopper), prosperous professional, youth, and empty nesters. You can view more on these at www.cbsoutdoor.co.uk. Audience segmentation strategies in a high risk drinkers campaign in the USA used software that mapped drinkers by demographic characteristic clusters and labelled these clusters as 'cyber millenials, laid back towners and city producers' (Moss et al. 2009). Other authors suggest that variables such as sensation seeking may be important in message design. D'Silva and Palmgreen (2007) examined anti-drug *Public Service Announcement*s (PSAs) and found that sensation-seeking target audiences have different media preferences. They recommend using design strategies and contexts that are high in sensation value. These examples suggest that there may be other characteristics of target groups that characterize the way they respond to messages, and messages should be tailored to these needs accordingly.

PSYCHOLOGICAL VARIABLES

Attitudes, beliefs and values

Campaigns often centre on the four variables of knowledge, attitude, beliefs and values. It is hypothesized that by changing these variables, we may be able to change aspects of health behaviour. These are also common variables in a range of theoretical health models (see Chapter 2) although it is important to define the differences between attitude, belief and values first before further discussion of this area.

An attitude is relatively stable, difficult to change, and inherently complex. Corcoran and Corcoran (2007) note that attitudes are made up of three components: cognitive, affective and conative. 'Cognitive' refers here to the individual evaluation of that attitude based on the information that person already has about that issue. 'Affective' refers to the likes and dislikes process of an attitude, rather like a weighing up process of pros and cons. 'Conative' refers to the behavioural intention towards the object or issue. Because attitudes are complex, they can sometimes result in contradictory behaviours. For example, a person could binge drink alcohol one evening (a behaviour) despite having a negative attitude (and disliking) the hangover in the morning (attitudes towards the behaviour).

A belief concerns the information that a person has about an object, for example, believing that tobacco can cause lung cancer. Health beliefs include what people believe might happen if they do (or do not) do something, such as a belief that cancer equates to death, or that physical activity increases longevity of life.

Values are usually acquired through the social world in which we live. Influential factors such as family and friends, religion or culture can impact on the values that we hold. In health the role of values tends to be seen in two ways. First, this may be seen in relation to how much value we attach to something. This could be the values we demonstrate such as stigmatising against someone who is unemployed if we believe that everyone should have a job and that anyone who does not work is lazy. Research indicates that the role of attitudes, beliefs and values on health is a complex one and most studies that have investigated these links have often centred their research on theoretical models (see chapter two).

Activity 4.7:   Attitudes, beliefs and values

Different people have different attitudes, beliefs, and values towards different health behaviours. Read the health behaviour description below and consider what different attitudes, beliefs and values the people listed *might* have towards these behaviours.

(Continued)

(Continued)

Health behaviour: *Reducing intake of foods high in fat including fried chicken, chips, crisps and other high fat foods.*

1   A 10-year-old girl.
2   A 60-year-old man who is overweight who has a number of chronic conditions including some heart complications.
3   A 40-year-old man who has type 2 diabetes.

Knowledge levels are also important in relation to health. It is important to be aware of the knowledge levels of your target group otherwise you may be telling them something they already know, or they may lack basic knowledge of the area you are focusing on. Do not assume just because a target group do (or do not) undertake health behaviours that they lack knowledge. For example, in the UK most people know that driving while using a mobile phone is illegal but a number of people still use their mobile phone this way and current campaigns in the UK aim to reduce this behaviour (see Chapter 8 for an example of this). This may suggest that knowledge levels may be high but a focus on attitudes, beliefs and values might be needed instead. Alternative strategies include increasing people's beliefs that using a mobile phone while driving can result in an accident, and promoting a more positive attitude to hands-free phones.

The role of knowledge may be important in health behaviours. For example, lower knowledge is associated with increased fear of TB (Hoa et al. 2009). Hoa et al. suggest that any educational programme needs to start with a clear 'understanding of the knowledge base of the target population and relate traditional beliefs and perceptions about the disease to modern knowledge' (2009: 11). This suggests that examining knowledge levels first may be a good place to start before examining beliefs (and from this, attitudes and values) about a health behaviour. Additional research has indicated that lack of knowledge is linked to an inability to undertake the behaviour. Karayurt et al. (2008) note that female high school students in their study report low levels of monthly breast self-examination. The most commonly cited reason for this was that they did not know how to perform a breast self-examination. A focus on knowledge of breast self-examinations would be an important component of a campaign to address this issue.

Some research indicates a clear link between knowledge, attitude and behaviour. For example, younger women in South Africa in a sample of women's knowledge, attitudes and behaviours to domestic and personal hygiene indicated that those with the most knowledge, and the most positive attitudes were more likely to perform preventive behaviours in relation to hygiene (Westaway and Viljkoen 2000). This is also the premise for some of the theoretical models described in Chapter 2 including the Theory of Planned Behaviour (Ajzen 1991).

Other theoretical models, such as the Health Belief Model (Becker 1974), consider the role of health beliefs to be important in changing health behaviours. Schouten et al. (2007) suggest that positive beliefs in adolescents about talking with parents on sexuality issues were positively associated with the amount of parent–adolescent sex communication. Gao et al. (2008) note that one of the most important factors in uptake of cervical screening is a belief that the tests are necessary. Beliefs do not always translate into behaviours, however. Byrd et al. (2004) found that young Hispanic women believed they were susceptible to cervical cancer and that screening was beneficial, but they did not attend screening. Chapter 5 also discusses the role of myths and beliefs.

Case study 4.3: Beliefs and infertility

Raine et al. (2003) found adolescents who believed they were infertile were significantly less likely to use any method of contraception, despite having not been confirmed medically infertile. In this study those who believed they were infertile were more likely to have mothers who had a first birth before 20, so there is a possibility that because they themselves were not pregnant at a young age, they believed themselves infertile. The study notes that this may have links to social definitions of fertility.

Activity 4.8: Beliefs and methods

You are designing a sexual health campaign for adolescent women based on Raine et al.'s (2003) findings in case study 4.3. The campaign aims to reduce rates of teenage pregnancy.

1   What sort of content would you have in your messages for this group that are linked to their beliefs?

Values can be more complex and are not generally represented in theoretical models in terms of a specific stage or step. In addition, they can be difficult to influence or change as they are not always observable. They may be influential in some health behaviours in particular, in addition to influencing attitudes and beliefs. They may also assert themselves through factors such as culture, religion or gender norms. Paek et al. (2008) in a study in Uganda found that in villages where more male-dominant and traditional gender roles were enforced, the less likely members of that village were to adopt family planning practices. This suggests that when patriarchal and male-dominated values are regarded as important and when they are maintained and conformed to (in countries like Uganda), they may have a strong influence on health. This includes elements such as women's roles inside and outside the home.

Additional psychological variables

Aside from the common psychological factors of attitudes, beliefs and values, a number of other variables may be influential in your target group. Variables such as self-efficacy, self-esteem, or peer pressure may also be important. There is a mixture of research to suggest variables such as self-efficacy may be important to health messages. Pluhar et al. (2008) state that in relation to mother–child sexual communication socio-economic variables are not associated with communication, but self-efficacy is. This may suggest that if an intervention is looking at increasing dialogue or communication around sexuality and communication, that it needs first to look at increasing self-efficacy. Lovell et al. (2007) note that in cervical cancer screening, factors such as shyness and embarrassment can be reasons why screening is not undertaken. This may also be the case in relation to other behaviours such as purchasing and using contraception. Research by Shahid et al. (2009) with Aboriginal Australians notes that factors such as fear of death, fatalism, shame and beliefs that cancer is contagious impact on decisions to access cancer services. As with social factors, therefore, a range of elements that could impact on psychological factors need to be considered in campaigns.

STRUCTURAL VARIABLES

Alongside social factors and psychological factors in health communication programmes, a number of structural variables may have an impact on health communication. Although one of the most common ways to define a target group is by age and sex, there are also a number of other structural variables that can be used. Boniface et al. (2001) note in a study on CHD-related behaviour that employment, type of housing and education were predictive of CHD-preventive behaviours. This indicates that there may be some links to structural factors and health communication programmes. In addition, location (e.g. inner city, urban, rural) may also be important. In China, one study found notable difference between rural and urban alcohol and cigarette behaviour with those living in rural areas more likely to engage in higher risk behaviours (Mao and Wu 2007). This study actually proposes that prevention efforts need to include not only gender, but also socio-economic status, place of residence and social environment. Chapter 3 considers location and settings for campaigns in more detail.

Case study 4.4:   Nutrition, physical activity and the wider environment

Lindsay et al. (2009) indicated that, in their research with immigrant Latino families in the USA, the factors that influence child feeding, diet and physical activity included supermarket proximity, food costs, neighbourhood safety and weather. They concluded that organization and environmental influences are important in these families.

DEFINING A TARGET GROUP

Previous chapters have drawn the reader's attention to important elements in planning campaigns and have highlighted some suggestions for choosing a target group. Once you have selected your target group then you need to map their main features. Figure 4.1 suggests a checklist of questions that you can ask about your target group. This is by no means a comprehensive list: you may be able to think of other variables that are important to your group depending on who they are. For example, country of birth, parental factors, societal roles or income levels might be important.

Figure 4.1 provides a list of social and structural factors to consider. They include questions of age and sex alongside demographic information about the group such as geography and education. Psychological factors include reference to knowledge, attitudes, beliefs and values in relation to the target group.

Factors	Possible questions to ask a target group
Social and structural	What is their age? What is their ethnicity? What is their sex? Do they have any religious/spiritual beliefs/philosophies? Are there any cultural points to note? What is their occupation? What are their education levels? What geographical area do they live in? Do they have access to the resources they may need for the health issue? Is location an important factor in performing the health behaviour? What are their knowledge levels of the health issue?
Psychological	What are their attitudes towards the health issue? What are their attitudes towards changing their behaviour? What beliefs do they hold about the health issue? What values do they hold about the health issue? What are their current behaviours in relation to the health issue?

Figure 4.1   Checklist of possible questions to ask target groups

---

Activity 4.9:   Identifying and defining a target group

1 Choose a target group (defined by a small age range, ethnicity and sex) and health issue of your choice and work through the target group checklist (Figure 4.1) to this issue answering each question in turn.
2 When you completed the checklist were there any questions that were difficult to answer?
3 What would you do to ensure that you could answer all the questions in the target group matrix effectively?

TAILORING INFORMATION

Tailoring information according to adapting a campaign to a specific group involves certain characteristics such as age, sex or ethnicity. This is based on the idea that interventions can be tailored to different behaviour change phases and characteristics of a target group (Tufano and Karras 2005). The process of tailoring requires selection of the determinants which influence the performance of health behaviour and then matching of the specific determinants to feedback for that group. Though the core programme content will be similar for different cultural groups, 'culturally appropriate examples, activities and printed materials should be designed specifically for each group' (Levy et al. 2004). Thus geographical and linguistic barriers may necessitate the delivery of slightly distinct programmes, although Levy does state that programmes can sometimes be successfully delivered to more than one group.

Woodrow et al. (2007), in their study on public perceptions of communicating information about bowel screening, note that flexible approaches to information provision that include perceptions of patients may be required. This study found some variations in type of information wanted for those eligible for bowel screening, for example, some wanted to minimize the negative aspects of screening, while others wanted all the information at the outset. In addition, some participants opposed the concept of providing balanced information to facilitate informed choice, instead preferring encouragement to participate in screening. Use of other characteristics such as geographical location has shown some success. Campo et al. (2008) note that adapting colorectal cancer information to a rural area in the USA by including elements such as images taken from a local festival and using local residents in the campaign demonstrated success.

Activity 4.10:   Tailoring information in practice

You are working on a campaign to promote awareness of testicular cancer. You are targeting men under 40 but need to tailor information specifically to different male beliefs. This means you have to provide different types of information and messages for different groups.
   What different messages could be influential with these people?

1 A 17-year-old black African male who believes that testicular cancer is something that happens to older people.
2 A 20-year-old white male who believes that testicular cancer is strongly associated with death.
3 A 38-year-old white male who believes that testicular cancer is a sexually transmitted infection and only contracted through unprotected sexual practices.
4 A 30-year-old Asian male who believes that testicular cancer is hereditary and therefore not a cancer he will contract.

To tailor information, a library of feedback messages or statements needs to be written. These should be based on a theoretical behavioural change model such as the Transtheoretical Model (Stages of Change model) (see Chapter 2). They are then coded using computer software or algorithms and merged into different documents to create different letters, leaflets or other similar printed materials. It is important to select determinants that have the potential to vary within individuals such as attitude or beliefs. It is neither cost-effective or necessary to choose homogeneous constructs (Halder et al. 2008). Gaps in data are also important as they may diminish the effectiveness of the tailored material (Halder et al. 2008). Computer software may be used for tailoring and this is discussed more in Chapter 5.

Case study 4.5: Tailoring campaigns to Chinese women

Sun et al. (2007) undertook a study to promote breast cancer practices in Chinese women in San Francisco. Two PSAs were created on breast cancer practices in English, Chinese and Mandarin. One was based on the American Cancer Association guidelines, the second on Breast Self-Examination (BSE) techniques. The study used Chinese media channels, including two major Chinese television stations, one Chinese radio station and two major Chinese newspapers.

The TV PSA was 30 seconds long and used three generations of women at a birthday party. The generations of women were associated with longevity and family harmony, and the emphasis was on BSE to promote these values. Over six months the PSA was aired 520 times on TV. Radio and newspaper also carried PSAs of the same themes over the six-month period.

When data in the streets of Chinatown was collected to demonstrate impact and effectiveness of the messages, a copy of a bilingual booklet about breast cancer screening was given to participants alongside a coin purse with breast health guidelines in Chinese.

HEALTH LITERACY

One final element that needs to be considered in the planning phases is health literacy. This refers to the capacity to locate and understand basic health information (Friedman and Hoffman-Goetz 2007). Health literacy also includes the notion that this information could be acted upon should the person wish. Kirksey et al. characterize health literacy as the 'ability to understand, and act correctly on health information' (2004: 91).

Health literacy is an area that is gradually receiving more attention in the health promotion literature. Nutbeam (2008) proposes that poor health literacy actually constitutes a risk factor for health. Health literacy has become more important as more people take on increased responsibility for their own health (Parker and Guzmararian 2003). It is essential that people are able to access the information they need in relation to health and make their own health decisions based on this information. For example, in medicine, you need knowledge to be able to participate fully in the treatment decision-making processes (Weintraub et al. 2004).

Research indicates that those with the greatest needs often have the poorest ability to understand health information (Parker and Gazmararian 2003). There can be a number of difficulties with written materials, for example, excessive information, high readability levels, lack of interactive features, and difficult or uncommon words (Doak et al. 1996). Literacy can increase with lower reading levels of materials and improved design characteristics, as well as the use of simple formats (Hoffman and McKenna 2006).

   There are a number of design steps that practitioners can work through to ensure that their materials can be read, understood, and acted upon by target groups. If all practitioners were able to review and design materials that were suited to their audiences, then health literacy problems would dramatically decrease. Chapter 6 describes the steps involved in designing resources effectively to improve the ability of end users to understand and comprehend health information. This element is something practitioners should consider in the planning phases as existing materials and resources may be inadequate for the target group.

CHAPTER REVIEW

This chapter has identified the role of age, sex, ethnicity, culture, and religion and spiritual beliefs in health promotion. It is clear that these social factors impact on each other and characteristics of a target group can rarely be focused on just one of these variables. In addition, the psychological variables of attitude, beliefs and values are important for health behaviours. Campaigns will need to consider a range of these social and psychological factors and how they impact on the target group. This chapter has considered the possible ways to tailor resources to culture alongside ways to tailor information to specific groups.

This chapter has:

- identified a range of social and psychological factors that make up or influence a target group;
- examined a range of variables that impact on the health of a target group aside from the standard social and psychological factors. The variables include different structural factors and health literacy;
- analysed the notion of tailoring materials to social characteristics such as culture to ensure materials are relevant to different target groups.

FURTHER READING

Corcoran, N and Corcoran, S (2007) Social and psychological factors in communication pp. 32–52 in Corcoran, N (ed.) *Communicating health strategies for health promotion* Sage, London.

Kreuter, M W, Lukwago, S N, Bucholtz, D C, Clark, E M and Sanders-Thompson,V (2002) Achieving cultural appropriateness in health promotion programs: targeted and tailored approaches. *Health Education and Behaviour* 30(2): 133–46.

5

Channels of communication

This chapter focuses on the various channels of health communication that can be used in campaigns. These include interpersonal, organizational and community channels. This chapter will consider different methods of communication in each of these channels including the use of experimental marketing, social marketing, mass media and information technology. It will also identify issues around timing of campaigns and the optimum exposure levels for campaigns.

This chapter aims to:

- explore channels of communication and highlight different strategies that can be used with each channel
- identify issues around timing of campaigns and increasing exposure of campaigns
- identify the uses of mass media, social marketing and information technology in campaigns and consider ways these can be utilized in practice.

CHANNELS

There are a variety of ways that messages can be communicated in health-related work. Message appeal depends on target audience characteristics and variables such as message exposure. Atkin (2001) suggests that health campaigns targeted at specific populations aim to have a modest impact, but this varies depending on different factors such as quality and quantity of messages as well as the current political and structural environment.

Health campaigns face stiff competition. More than ten years ago Kraak and Pelletier (1998) noted in the USA that one large fast food chain delivered more than 200 advertisements annually and used a multifaceted sales approach. Globally they were sponsors of sporting events. Locally they targeted different ethnic young people through radio and Cable TV stations. Sub-populations such as mothers were targeted with bilingual messages, newsletters and promotions. Inside the restaurant toy 'give-aways', scratch cards and placemat games were available. Though this information is more than ten years old, it highlights the competition health campaigns will face, as in reality not many health campaigns will be able to rival the strengths of these marketing techniques. Health campaigns therefore have considerable work to do to ensure that their messages are heard above health-damaging ones. Possible solutions include ensuring appropriate channels of communication are used alongside the use of a variety of media strategies (rather than just one) in campaigns.

SELECTING CHANNELS OF COMMUNICATION

Health campaign designers have a host of potential media sources. The medium chosen in a campaign impacts on how information is processed, assimilated and recalled (Bryne and Curtis 2000). The choice of channels of communication therefore requires careful thought. One of the fundamental questions is: which source can be used the most effectively and efficiently with the biggest potential outcomes? There are different communication infrastructures in different communities (Wilkin and Ball-Rokeach 2006), and they will all be used differently by target audiences. Atkin (2001) recommends exploring a diverse range of sources in campaign efforts. Essentially the nature of the message and the media used should be shaped by consideration of both the communicator and the audience (Peattie 2007).

To identify channels of communication, it helps to divide them into three groups, all of which will be examined in this chapter (Table 5.1). These three groups are:

- interpersonal/intrapersonal (individual communication one-to-one);
- organizations (such as schools);
- community (such as billboard or newspaper advertising).

Each type of channel has a part to play in campaigns. Research suggests that there may be a need to include more than one of these categories to increase effectiveness and reach of campaigns.

Table 5.1   Examples of the three channels of communication

Type of channel	Definition of the channel	Examples of each channel
Interpersonal	Individual communication one-to-one	Health practitioner to patient/client, parent to child
Organizations	Locations where people live, work and play	Schools, workplaces, universities, supermarkets, places of worship or leisure centres
Community	Wider media and wider community structures	Mass media channels, political or structural channels

---

Activity 5.1:   Different channels of communication

Look at the following website for the Department of Health (2009) Change4Life campaign: www.nhs.uk/change4life

1 How many different channels of communication are mentioned as being used on this website?
2 Do these channels cover all the categories as mentioned in Table 5.1?

Use of multiple channels is considered the best way to reach health communication goals. A number of authors suggest this (Atkin 2001; Bessinger et al. 2004; Corcoran 2007a; Tones and Green 2004). This is deemed important in particular for behaviour change messages that may need to look at a variety of change variables, such as knowledge and attitude, as well as behaviour (Bessinger et al. 2004). As behavioural change theories, in particular, are criticized for their individualistic approach and their dismissal of wider structural factors (Dutta-Bergman 2005), it is essential that more than one channel (especially a mix of wider media and interpersonal channels) is used to counteract this problem. The highly publicized and researched social marketing VERB™ campaign in the USA used multiple channels to promote its goal of increasing physical activity with teens aged 9–13. They had two strategies that used both large-scale media use with low personal involvement and tactics to reach smaller audiences with high personal involvement. Tones and Green (2004) propose mass media should not be used on its own but alongside interpersonal interaction. Chapter 8 outlines a range of campaigns that use multi-media channels.

Several factors need to be considered when choosing a communication channel. They include: ability to reach the audience; style preferences; accessibility; and cost. Understanding channel availability and reliability is important as different channels have different consequences for knowledge and behaviour (Buckley et al. 2008). There is a shortage of research findings to demonstrate which channels are the most effective (Cunningham et al. 1999). This might be because channel effectiveness differs considerably by target group and topic and there are few consistencies between campaigns using similar topics but different audiences. Buckley et al. (2008) considers that linguistic, cultural, religious barriers and marital status can impact on information channels used.

In addition, there are differences in sub-groups. For example, Artienza et al. (2006) examined different subgroups of people who have similar levels of inactivity. Each group has different defining characteristics which could be used in channel selection – for example some watch more television, and others read newspapers or are more likely to access the internet. It may be logical therefore to choose a selection of channels to take into account these differences.

Activity 5.2:   Identifying sub-groups

1   Consider different people (for example, children, teenagers, adults) who eat foods that are high in fat. What reasons might they give for eating a diet that is high in fat?
2   Are they all likely to use the same sources of information for health advice? Why/ why not?

The number of channels to be used in a campaign will depend on the audience. Bessinger et al. (2004) note that the likelihood of ever having used a condom increased with the number of media channels cited. Duerksen et al. (2005) consider that the doctrine of marketing is that multiple messages must be received to achieve high levels of awareness. This would suggest that a range of channels may need to be used to achieve this. Even in small-scale campaigns, two or more channels could feasibly be used from the same category. Factors including volume of information, repetition of messages, placement and scheduling of messages also need consideration (Atkin 2001). Choosing a channel is important, but then how the channel is used in a campaign is also integral to the campaign.

Media channels need to be selected carefully. A lack of access will mean that messages cannot be received by the target audience. In addition, if access is available, the assumption should not be that health messages are appropriate for these channels. Kari (2006) notes that in rural Nigeria a large proportion of the population do not have access to the internet, television or radio and thus oral tradition is prevalent due in part to high illiteracy rates. This study does suggest, however, that media such as television may be accessed through friends and family, so although ownership of these media sources is small, they may still reach a larger number of people. In this study, however, television was seen as a source of entertainment and propaganda and might not be suitable for health messages. This is not to say that television as a media source should be ruled out. For example, one solution could be the adoption of an 'edutainment' soap opera or serial which combines entertainment with education and encourages interpersonal discussion.

This would link the source (television) with the purpose of watching television (a social occasion with friends and family) with oral traditions (discussions with friends and family).

Edutainment using soap operas and serials has produced some promising findings in some contexts. In Ethiopia, a radio soap opera-style drama focusing on modern family planning demonstrated some success (Farr et al. 2005), and in South Africa the 'Soul City' (Soul City Institute 2009) education-entertainment utilizes radio dramas as part of their overall campaign strategy. You can find more information about Soul City at www.soulcity.org.za.

INTERPERSONAL COMMUNICATION

Interpersonal communication is communication between individuals, such as mother to daughter, or peer to peer. Families, friends, peers and medical or health professionals are a strong source of health information. Different target groups rely on family and friends more or less, depending on the group. For example, members of multi-generational families may have more access to health information via the family (Buckley et al. 2008)

The use of friends and family to promote health is an interesting issue. Many campaigns advisors now propose that promoting interpersonal discussion to help change attitudes, social norms, or behaviours is important. Women tend to report the importance of friends and family more than men, for example, more women than men reported friends and family as being important for TB knowledge in Vietnam (Hoa et al. 2009). In addition, some ethnic groups rely more on interpersonal communication for health information. Cunningham et al. (1999) note that lower education black groups are more likely to use friends and family, as well as religious sources. Oetzel (2007) also considers that key cultural variables are associated with communication preferences: he notes some Hispanic cultural values promote communication with friends and family. Children may also consider friends and family an important source of health information. Gray et al. (2005) found that despite the internet being a primary source of information for health, peers and adults still remain important.

Research has suggested that this type of communication may be more influential than the use of mass media. For example, a study in Belize (Central America) of a malaria control programme found that interpersonal communication in a community had more influence on behaviour change than media (e.g. sign, poster and pamphlet) (Cropley 2004). Although the study acknowledged some study design flaws, it concluded that malaria control programs should understand malaria knowledge, attitudes, perceptions and treatment behaviours of individuals and communities in the design of messages.

One of the strengths of interpersonal communication is that it may be more responsive than media efforts to individual characteristics. However, most campaigns do not rely on interpersonal communication. This is because of the high cost and low reach of such methods. However, campaigns may include elements of interpersonal communication, such as telephone help-lines, or mobile phone short messaging services (SMS), embedded in a campaign that could increase elements of interpersonal communication. For example, alongside email, telephone and text support there is a 'Frankbot' on the TalktoFrank (2009a) drugs website http://talktofrank.com/ available 24/7 on MSN messenger.

Activity 5.3:   Including interpersonal elements

You are working on a campaign to increase the number of males being screened for prostate cancer.

1   What interpersonal elements could you include in your campaign?
2   How much time, money or resources might these consume?

There are several ways in which friends or family networks can be involved in campaigns. Encouraging dialogue and discussion in health campaigns within these networks can help to engage a community with health issues. Research by Aubel et al. (2004) in Senegal found that grandmothers can promote good maternal and child health practices in pregnant women as older and more experienced women play an important role in health of the family. In a community setting Victor et al. (2009) report on the design of a study that will use barbers to offer a blood pressure check with each haircut. The barbers will also encourage medical referral if necessary, as well as using real-life customers modelling ideal behaviours. Delvin (2008) notes in a newspaper article that campaigns that are more personal and that use friends and family may be more effective than mass campaigns. This article gives the example of Jamie Oliver (a celebrity chef in the UK) and the workings of his restaurant where local people come and learn to cook and then pass these skills on to friends and family. The result is that local people feel empowered and in turn assist others with cooking skills.

NARRATIVE COMMUNICATION

>>

Recently, there has been interest in the use of stories to promote health. *Narrative* is the main way that people communicate with each other every day. Although the evidence base is small, it is possible to suggest that an audience may view narrative communication as more personally believable and memorable than non-narrative forms (Hinyard and Kreuter 2007). Narrative communication includes entertainment-education, story telling, testimonials and other stories. Hinyard and Kreuter define narrative communication as 'any cohesive and coherent story ... that provides information about scene, characters and conflict; raises unanswered questions ... and provides resolution' (2007: 778). They note five different types of stories and these can all be applied and used in health communication.

- Official stories are one version of an event.
- Invented stories are a fictional account.
- First-hand stories are the retelling of a story by the first person.
- Second-hand stories are the retelling of a story heard (or read about) by someone else.
- Culturally common stories are stories that are general or pervasive in a cultural environment.

In the context of health, an official story could consist of a story in a newspaper that relates to health. Invented stories could be soap operas or fictional characters in a health situation. A first-hand story could come from a health practitioner giving guidance, and a second-hand one from someone who has been advised by a health practitioner and is passing knowledge on (i.e. mother to daughter regarding care of a baby). Commonly recited stories or tales could be re-worked to include factually correct information, e.g. how diarrhoeal disease is transmitted.

Wilkin and Ball-Rokeach (2006) suggest that stories form part of a neighbourhood and community structure and that health educators or change agents need to become part of this story network. They consider that ethnic media needs to integrate health stories that are relevant to their audience and instigate interpersonal storytelling. This might have the advantage of allowing health to become part of the story network, not something that is outside of this. In addition, Tones and Green (2004) suggest that the use of media such as soap operas or edutainment may be amenable to fostering health promotion.

Wilkin and Ball-Rokeach (2006) consider that health stories need to be framed in a way that encourages interpersonal discussion rather than just providing facts and statistics. They note, for example, celebrities with health problems often provoke interpersonal discussion and information seeking. For example, when a celebrity in the UK (Jade Goody) was diagnosed with cervical cancer and subsequently died, the number of women screened for cervical cancer increased dramatically in the UK (Sturcke 2009; Elliott 2009). Although exact figures are still unknown, this public interest in cervical cancer has been nicknamed the 'Jade Goody effect'. Other celebrities engage in events such as 'Movember' (The Prostate Cancer Charity 2009) where men are encouraged to grow a moustache to support prostate cancer (see www.movember.com for more information).

One problem is that stories, including myths and rumours, are not always true and so can in fact enforce health-*damaging* behaviours. Ma et al. (2008) identify a number of myths and misconceptions in smoking in China including the belief that the dangers of smoking are not severe and can be controlled. Wynn et al. (2009) also suggest that emails sent to a reproductive health website indicate that sexual health misconceptions and myths are formed from abstinence only programs in the USA, media confusion, inaccurate websites and terminology used in health campaigns. One role of a campaign could then be to work with these stories or myths. This might ensure that you include correct and appropriate terminology in your campaign messages. In addition, you might address myths in your campaign materials. For example, Thesite.org (2009), a young person's guide to life, includes sexual health myths as part of its sex and relationships section. Kaler (2009) notes the large number of rumours that have persisted in

Africa over the years about vaccines (for example, polio vaccines or vitamin tablets) and the links to sterility that persist in some cultural groups. If these stories are recognized, then practitioners can work with the existing stories to promote health more effectively.

Activity 5.4:   Working with myths

Alcorn (2005) notes that a number of myths around TB are still barriers to screening and treatment in many countries. Some of these myths include the following:

- TB is incurable.
- TB causes impotence.
- TB treatment kills.
- TB equals AIDS, and therefore all TB patients have AIDS and will die.

1   How might you address these in a campaign?
2   What sort of messages might you design to address these myths?
3   What media sources could you use to effectively address these myths?

ORGANIZATIONAL COMMUNICATION

Different organizations influence health in different ways. These organizations generally include large organizations such as schools or workplaces and smaller organizations such as youth groups, places of worship or sporting organizations. Chapter 3 discusses settings in more detail and how these can be used in campaigns. The communication networks within organizations can be influential in health, and although most documentation focuses on the more traditional settings of schools or workplaces, there is also a place for smaller organisations such as places of worship. Faith organizations, for example, have been found to be influential in health, partly due to their strong support networks (Duan et al. 2005). Locations that reach different ethnic minority groups may also be important. Wilkin and Ball-Rokeach (2006) note that campaign designers often fail to consider the potential of ethnic media for high-risk groups and consider that ethnic media play an integral role in a community infrastructure. Their study noted that Latinos found that interpersonal communication with friends, family or health professionals followed by ethnic television were the most important for health. This suggests possible different information sources as opposed to mainstream communication sources.

COMMUNITY COMMUNICATION

Community communication is a wide-ranging concept. It includes wider communication structures that reach whole communities, including mass media, such as television and radio, and information technology. In addition, other strategies such as *experimental marketing* may also fall under this heading. Practitioners use a range of these strategies.

Mass media

Mass media is the term applied to resources that can be distributed without personalisation. Mass media can be divided into four categories (Corcoran 2007a) as follows:

1 audio-visual broadcast media including television and radio;
2 audio-visual non-broadcast media including videos, CDs or tapes;
3 print media, including newspapers, magazines, leaflets or booklets;
4 electronic media (or information technology), including internet, mobile phones or computer packages.

This chapter will consider media from all four categories. Impacts from mass media use alone tend to be low as people are lost at each stage of the message (Atkin 2001) and thus the impact of mass media campaigns alone can be quite small. Research suggests that there may be effective uses of mass media in health, for example, the use of mass media can be instrumental in promoting condom use to prevent STIs (Bessinger et al. 2004).

However, the best way to use media is still disputed and a number of authors have debated its relative advantages and disadvantages (see Corcoran 2007a). Tones and Green (2004) suggest four possible effective uses of media in health. These include: (1) gaining unpaid advertising (for example, through providing newsworthy information); (2) agenda setting in health issues; (3) consciousness raising (for example, of a disease); and (4) critical consciousness raising (for example, regarding a social issue). Mass media has different characteristics – it can be high reach (such as television) or low reach (such as magazines).

Activity 5.5:   Effective uses of media

Consider the four different effective uses of media as highlighted by Tones and Green (2004).

- Gaining unpaid advertising such as newsworthy information.
- Agenda setting in health issues.
- Consciousness raising, for example, of a disease.
- Critical consciousness raising such as a social issue.

1 Think about mass media campaigns that you have seen and give one example for all four of Tones and Green's points.

It has been argued that mass media has a variety of effects on knowledge, attitude, and behaviour. The relationships are complex and effects reported are generally small for mass media when used in isolation. Dobbinson et al. (2008) note that greater SunSmart advertising exposure was significantly associated with respondents' skin cancer prevention attitudes and behaviours, although the effects were much weaker without the community and environmental changes such as locally-based campaign work. This may suggest that there are benefits of combining interpersonal communication with mass media efforts, and current research seems to suggest that this may have the most effective impact.

Television

Television is the medium most consistently cited as the main source of information for most groups in the Western world over the past decade or more. Older academic sources typically suggest television, followed by news and print media, were the most frequently used sources of HIV/AIDS information and showed little variation between ethnicity, age and education, although other sources such as interpersonal sources do show differences (Cunningham et al. 1999). Kraak and Pelletier (1998) suggest television is the medium that provides the widest reach for young children. More recent research indicates a similar trend. Hoa et al. (2009) note that the most common source of TB knowledge was television and Porto (2007) found that television is seen as the most effective medium to reach people in a condom use campaign. Li et al. (2009) also note that television is one of the main sources of HIV information and Tilson et al. (2004) suggest TV is perceived as the most effective route of STI knowledge in young people.

Although television is cost effective in large campaigns due to its high reach (Li 2009), the medium does have considerable limitations, especially cost. DuRant et al. (2006) note that the weaknesses of television are cost, limited effectiveness, and the influence of competing priorities. This might mean that television will not be the main media source used for many small-scale campaigns. However, there are other visual channels such as *YouTube* (www.youtube.com) that can be utilized for free and which provide high visual impact opportunities. YouTube is currently being used in a range of new campaigns. Chapter 8 provides examples of these.

Magazines and newspapers

The potential for promotion of health in magazines and newspapers is not well reported. Atkin (2001) considers that public relation techniques such as news stories and features are often under-used in campaigns. This is surprising given that research in the UK suggests that the time spent reading an average magazine is 30 minutes, and that 61 per cent of readers read for 30 minutes or more (National Readership Survey (NRS) 2009). Weekly newspapers are read on average for 40 minutes each day (NRS 2009). Although readerships may be small for specific newspapers, which may limit the reach of messages, the time spent reading magazines and newspapers suggests that many people have time to consider what they are reading. There is also evidence to suggest that magazines that are read may be able to incorporate some messages easily into their standard material. Research suggests that supermarket magazines have a high readership (NRS 2009), which would suggest that issues centred on healthy eating, alcohol, coronary heart disease or other lifestyle connected issues could be integrated into these publications fairly easily.

There are a number of ways in which health issues can be integrated into magazines and newspapers, aside from advertising. Clements et al. (2006) suggest four general styles of health-related topics in men's magazines which relate to magazines and newspapers in general. These are:

- general health and lifestyle stories;
- medical issues, for example, advice or therapies;
- letters to an expert, for example, doctors;
- letters to an agony aunt with health content.

Potentially any of these could be used in campaigns, although the first source may be the most likely choice for health professionals. A fifth could be added, namely advertisements, for example, advertising local stop smoking services or giving information or raising awareness about a range of health issues.

A few studies have noted other opportunities to promote health in newspapers and magazines. These include Clements et al. (2006), who suggest that men's readership of women's magazines is high and possible messages directed at men in these magazines could be increased. Harrison and Bond (2007) suggest that the popularity of gaming magazines with pre-pubescent boys for leisure is also high, and current magazines often expose readers to hyper-muscular unrealistic body types with racial disparities in role models, particularly as African-American readership is high. These represent missed opportunities and both magazines and newspapers should be considered as ways to use media to promote positive health.

Activity 5.6: Using magazines to promote health

You are working on a campaign to increase positive self-image and self-esteem in an ethnic minority group in your local area.

1 Identify which magazines this group may read.
2 What different ways could you promote your aim in these magazines?

Generating media-worthy news is also important in a campaign: the resulting *news items* may reach different audiences or reinforce the message amongst those the campaign is aimed at. Writing press releases, news stories and generating coverage of issues at local level should be part of any health campaign. It is important to remember that newspapers are often read daily and messages may need more repetition over time.

>>

Other mass media

Other common sources of mass media information include public service announcements (PSA), radio, billboards, posters, leaflets, newspapers, magazines and other paper-based sources. These have had varying degrees of success and research findings can be contradictory or sparse. For example, PSAs have been associated with some success in the USA. Sun et al. (2007) note that repeated PSA viewing of two different breast cancer announcements (one newspaper and one radio) were associated with increased knowledge and practice of breast cancer prevention. In the UK, recent attention has been drawn to a You-Tube PSA designed to prevent texting on a mobile phone while driving. This has received much publicity although the impact of this is not yet known. Chapter 8 provides more detail.

Bessinger et al. (2004) considered radio the most effective channel with the greatest audience reach: there was a strong relationship between exposure, condom knowledge and use of condoms and radio messages. Research indicates that the most responsive audience to radio is the 18–34 age range (Rajar 2009), suggesting potential for health messages aimed at a younger audience.

Leaflets are one of the most common print media. Leaflets have been found to increase knowledge (Dyer et al. 2005). Other researchers have examined leaflets and note they increase knowledge but not awareness (Petti and Scully 2007). Larger media sources such as bus wraps and billboards are also used in campaigns, but rarely alone and therefore the impact of these is rarely noted. Bus wraps are seen to have some beneficial effects such as large-scale mobility and high visibility (CBS outdoor 2009c). Billboards have received some success but research has produced contradictory findings. For example, billboards were considered the least effective in reaching people in research by Porto (2007) for promoting condom use, although were associated with more supportive norms for buying condoms.

It has been suggested that written formats that are minimally distracting may be more effective in increasing knowledge than active channels such as visual or audio means (Bryne and Curtis 2000). Research by Pinfold (1999) also suggests there is a strong correlation between passive channels of printed media such as stickers, posters and leaflets and higher knowledge scores for hand washing and dishwashing behaviours. Porto (2007) notes some contradictory findings from the 'carnival campaign' in Brazil that suggest television and billboards were associated with more supportive norms for buying condoms and posters provoked a negative effect norm for purchasing condoms. The study notes that the reasons are as yet uncertain.

Each of these media sources has different potential for health campaigns and the relative advantages need to be considered when choosing which media source to use. Generally a search of the literature on the media source that is intended for use will elicit a list of pros and cons. For example, billboards are generally located in geographically targeted locations, they have repetitive value, are physically dominating and are cost effective (DuRant et al. 2006).

They are also limited, however, by the fact that messages or images need to be simple and easy to interpret. Furthermore, only those who own cars or travel that route via public transport or those resident in that area will view the message.

Activity 5.7: Advantages and disadvantages of using different media

You are working on a health campaign that aims to reduce the stigma of mental illness in your local community. You want to use two mass media resources.

1 What are the advantages and disadvantages of using billboards, local newspapers, leaflets and a radio advertisement in your local area?

The use of mass media does not necessarily mean there should be just one message for everyone: media messages still need to be tailored to their intended audience(s). For example, in an exercise video in a workplace physical activity intervention that is aimed at sedentary, overweight adults, the leader of the video is a mature, overweight non-athletic black woman (Yancey et al. 2004). The videos were made in English and Spanish, with music, graphics and people represented in the video tailored to the audience.

Information technology

Information technology (IT) is sometimes referred to as 'new media'. Its use has grown considerably in the past ten years or so. It has been argued that new media channels are best used to augment or complement media use rather than replace these sources (Tian and Robinson 2008). This does depend on the campaign strategy and aims, as in some instances the use of traditional media might not be appropriate. The internet has been found to have a powerful influence on health (Evers et al. 2003) and it has been argued that IT is an ideal medium to effect behaviour change as technology is integrated into many aspects of society (Marcus et al. 2000). The potential of the internet to promote health may not have been fully realized (Peattie 2007) and research in this area in health campaigns is ongoing.

The internet has a number of potential uses for health communication. Some studies demonstrate that internet-based communication can be successful in achieving behaviour change. Hunter et al. (2008) found that in an internet-based weight management study, participants achieved weight loss and prevented additional weight gain. Increasingly, websites contain more interactive elements to increase user engagement, for example, the Trident website (Trident 2009a) encourages you to roll your mouse over an image of a police cell. If you roll your mouse over a picture, it says 'Photo of your girlfriend. But she won't be by the time you get out.' Or the toilet which says 'No seat, no privacy. No idea who's been using it.' You can see more at www.stoptheguns.org/. Similar techniques are used on the TalktoFrank website (2009b), where you are encouraged to 'have a drag on a spliff' to then see what can happens. See http://talktofrank.com/cannabis.aspx for more information. Other interactive elements such as discussion boards and message boards are also found on health-related websites, for example, Cancer Research UK (2009) run a message board called 'CancerChat' available at www.cancerchat.org.uk/.

Peattie (2007) notes six possible advantages of using information technology in health communication. These include the notion of empowerment, the maintenance of long-term relationships, customizability, immediate impact, interconnectivity and confidentiality. Table 5.2 outlines these six areas with an explanation and example of these in practice. For example, empowerment can be linked to the individual ability to choose information or ask questions about health topics. In health, this might take the form of searching for health information on a website or asking a question to an expert through an 'ask a question' function.

Table 5.2   Information technology uses in health information

	Explanation of terminology	Example of the use in a health campaign
Empowerment	Individuals choose which information they want and when	Emails or discussion boards can encourage participation
Long-term retention	Target groups can return many times to use resources	Websites can be long-term or CD ROMs can be re-used over long period of time
Customizability	Tailored messages or feedback can be given or information found can be specific to a group	Individual emails or tailored responses to quizzes can be given
Immediacy	Location of information or feedback can be immediate	Questions may have automatically generated answers that provide an immediate response
Interconnectivity	Interaction between people or providers with no barriers i.e. age or location	Communication can be facilitated through a discussion board or social networking devices i.e. Twitter
Confidentiality	Allows people to access information or ask questions without saying who they are	Questions can be posted anonymously

Activity 5.8:   Adapting information technology for campaigns

You are working on a campaign to promote community and neighbourhood safety in your local area. One part of your campaign includes a website.

1   Choose any three of the categories in Table 5.2 and consider how you could build these elements into a health website.

One area that has received attention recently is the use of information technology for tailoring messages. Suggs (2006) considers that information technology lends itself better than print-based materials to tailoring information. Suggs and McIntyre (2009) note that online communication should be tailored to be effective as this can enhance the efficacy of health communication. As this area is still developing, they offer a number of questions for developing and evaluating online tailored communication including what kind of variables are needed to tailor effectively and what channels should be used for feedback delivery. Matching materials correctly is seen as the main key to successful tailoring (De Nooijer et al. 2002).

Another growing area in health communication is the use of short messaging service (SMS) through mobile phones. Atun and Sittampalam (2006) note three main advantages of SMS including efficiency gains in delivery of healthcare, benefits to the patient and benefits to public health. In relation to the last advantage this may mean sending health promotion information via SMS to different target groups as part of a campaign. Fjeldsoe et al. (2009) note that most studies centre on clinical care with a limited number of high quality studies centring on behaviour change. There is some suggestion that there are positive behaviour changes associated with SMS but these are small and difficult to substantiate due to different measures. There are examples of SMS being used in campaigns in different ways. For example, the London Metropolitan police (2009) asked young people the question 'Which issues should your SNT tackle? You Decide: The groups, the dark alley or the journey?' (SNT is a safer neighbourhood's team). They encouraged young people to text their answers, or use *Bebo* to gain views. This campaign can be viewed at www.met.police.uk/campaigns/you_decide/you_decide.htm

Future developments in the use of information technology may include the use of entertainment websites or online worlds, as well as games consoles. In relation to games consoles, Nintendo Wii users can now access packages such as 'Wii Fit' aimed at increasing personal fitness levels. Different research projects are looking at using Wii for other purposes such as rehabilitation. Virtual worlds such as 'Secondlife' may be a possibility in health-related work, for example, virtual health centres or health promotion advice clinics could be set up. In addition websites such as online game sites or music and entertainment sites such as YouTube could be used to promote health. The British Heart Foundation '2 minutes' video (BHF 2008) (see Chapter 8) is also available on YouTube (see www.youtube.com) alongside other campaigns.

Social networking sites, such as Facebook, Bebo, Twitter and MySpace, may also have potential for health-related communication. Waters et al. (2009) note ways that non-profit organizations use Facebook to promote participation and social networking. In New Zealand a metal health suicide prevention Twitter site was launched in 2009 and is run by SPINZ (Suicide Prevention in New Zealand) (2009). You can view this at www.twitter.com/suicidenz. It is also worth noting that sites do not necessarily need to be health-specific to have the potential to promote health, news sites or young people's magazine or music sites may all have health promotion potential.

The use of information technology also has a number of disadvantages. These include over-use of IT, the location of health-damaging information, isolation, and the misinterpretation of information (Peattie 2007). Also the digital divide is still evident: not all groups can access information technology and some therefore have restricted access to these information formats. Peattie (2007) also notes that simply having a presence on the internet (through a website) does not automatically equate to success, and Waters et al. (2009) make a similar point in relation to Facebook. A number of design features need to be included, such as using credible sources and interactive features (see Corcoran 2007a), and websites need to be promoted and evaluated to ensure success.

Experimental marketing

One approach that has received more attention in recent years is the use of experimental marketing. Experimental marketing is the use of different types of marketing as an experiment to see whether they work. It is generally recommended that these do not form the main strategy for an intervention, but instead complement other strategies. Noar et al. (2009) note in HIV campaigns the use of strategies such as baseball cards, postcards, condom packets and interpersonal strategies such as peer education and skill building workshops. Figure 5.1 is an example of a pair of cardboard glasses distributed at festivals and used in a DfT (2009b) drug driving campaign with the message 'Drug driving: your eyes will give you away' (see Chapter 8 for more on this campaign).

The VERB™ campaign used event sponsorship with 'activity zones', street teams with 'ambassadors' who had unique performance skills, 'any tour' mobile

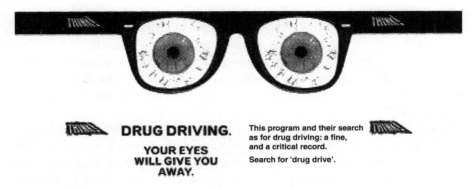

Figure 5.1　Drug driving: your eyes will give you away glasses
Source: DfT (2009).

trucks that set themselves up at amusement parks and gave out 'yellow balls' to use in schools in communities with the VERB™ brand (see Heitzler et al. 2008, for more information). Their use of unconventional ways of performing promotional activities with few resources was referred to as 'guerrilla marketing'. The street ambassadors who used skills like break-dancing to promote physical activity are considered an example of guerrilla marketing.

Case study 5.1: Experimental marketing in the VERB™ campaign

The VERB™ campaign 2002–6 promoted physical activity in *'tweens'* aged 9–13 and placed emphasis on having fun and breaking rules in a sporting context. One strategy was the invention of a game called 'cross over' that aims to combine two sports together to create a new game. Schools received a kit (or downloaded resources from the website below) for this. The kit included: a teacher guide, educator letter, parent letters, two posters, dry erase laminated poster for results, award certificates, an interactive games wheel to suggest games to play and prizes such as inflatable balls and rubber bracelets. Other resources included materials and resources for activities such as 'play without borders', 'anytime doubletime', 'action awards', 'action appreciation day', 'make it up' and 'yellow ball'.

>>

See CDC (2009) www.cdc.gov/youthcampaign/index.htm for resources and more information and Heitzler et al. (2008) for a review of these experimental marketing techniques. Chapter 8 also has an overview of the VERB™ campaign.

Activity 5.9: Experimental marketing

1 Identify one group and one health issue in your community and one setting where you could undertake experimental marketing as part of your campaign.
2 What different marketing strategies could you use with your group to engage them in the health issue?

Experimental marketing – the use of theatre

Research suggests that the use of theatre may have potential in campaigns to promote health. Mbizvo (2006) notes that theatre has the potential to promote and reinforce health messages, as illustrated through a range of examples of theatre in Africa. Mbizvo states that, in places of low literacy and few interpersonal conversations about HIV, theatre can help to demystify issues and barriers to communication around HIV. In the UK the most popular use of theatre is generally theatre in education and therefore in schools. Starkey and Orme (2001) discuss a primary school drug drama project aimed at attitudes, choices and decisions around legal and illegal drugs. It is disappointing that generally theatre tends only to be reported in schools as there is potential in a range of communities to use theatre as part of a health campaign.

There are a range of dramatic techniques that could be used in health campaigns. One of the advantages of theatre in education is that some techniques can be used to foster two-way communication and enable people to represent their own interpretation of health issues. Mbizvo (2006) notes that after one play there was a question and answers session, and this material was subsequently worked into future productions. Sawney (2006) suggests seven techniques that can be used to promote health and a number of these could be possible campaign components. Street theatre, where an issue-based scene is performed in public spaces to stimulate discussion or interest, is similar to the experimental marketing techniques used in VERB™ (see case study 5.1). Elements such as forum theatre (where action is 'frozen' and the drama discussed), monologues (one-way communication) or truth seating, where members of the audience can ask questions to people in 'role', could also form parts of a communication campaign. See case study 5.2 for an example of theatre use in education.

Case study 5.2: 'Facefront' theatre in education

In the UK a number of theatre in education groups exist. One of these is 'Facefront'. A number of plays have been written by this group:

- 'Opening the can' which is about the emotional and physical journey of a family with cancer.
- 'Unique recipe 2' centred on the relationship between healthy mind and body with a focus on obesity.
- 'Sex FM' an interactive theatre on sexual health issues for young people.

For more information on these, see Facefront (2009) available at www.facefront.org.

There are some similarities between experimental marketing and social marketing. Essentially, social marketing uses a selection of promotional tools and materials matched to customer preference based on the four Ps framework (Thackery et al. 2007). By matching customer preferences with the four Ps, a promotion strategy is created. Social marketing concepts and planning models were considered in Chapter 1. However, mass media cannot be considered without reference to social marketing. Social marketing is the application of marketing to health with the acknowledgement of economics, legal issues and policy (Tones and Green 2004).

There have been a range of successful campaigns that include social marketing. The successful US 'Truth' campaign launched in 2000 aimed to build a teen brand that appeals to young people to compete with tobacco brands. It used negative advertising to promote an alternative to cigarette brands (see, for example, Apollonio and Malone 2009; Evans et al. 2002).

TIME

Exactly when campaigns should occur and how long they should last are important, but little understood, issues. Although all planned campaigns will have a time frame to work to, achieving optimal targeting of a campaign can be difficult. Research from the field of marketing suggests that the correct timing for a promotional mass media campaign is uncertain (Delre et al. 2007). Delre et al. note that timing is crucial and can be aided by utilizing different networks of consumers. Advertising too soon and too strongly can result in low market penetration: advertising too late means that people will have moved on. Thus groundwork may need to be undertaken in health campaigns before the final launch of the biggest part of the campaign. This ensures optimum reach of the target group.

One suggestion is that the target group should not only be involved in the planning of campaigns, but should also be targeted before the launch of the main campaign event. This might be advertising a local service or distributing flyers or leaflets before a big event or the launch of a new radio or newspaper campaign. This practice is similar to promotional advertising before the launch of a new music album or a new film in the cinema, for example, actors or musicians do talk shows, radio slots, magazine shots, and so on and the audience is therefore made aware of the 'product' before it is launched. Fast food chains often exploit new cinema events and they promote materials such as badges, balloons, toys and give-aways inside restaurants before a film launch. Health campaigns should be aiming for something similar. Although the behaviour might already be known (for example, most people know that they should not smoke), the campaign strategy needs to be unique enough to engage audiences with old messages.

Some research suggests that the length of a campaign and the number of messages it transmits may be important variables. Greater programme exposure and engagement are associated with enhanced sun protection (Andreeva et al. 2008). Dobbinson et al. (2008), in an evaluation of the SunSmart campaign in Australia, note that long-term commitment is needed to health issues such as sun safety, as trends (such as fashions for suntans, or the current growth of indoor tanning centres) can change. Such health communication efforts will need to respond to these new challenges. Ruel et al. (2008) note in behaviour change campaigns for maternal and child health that longer programme exposure is linked to greater effects. Atkin (2001) considers that there can be maximum saturation and that campaigns need to aim for moderate repetition. Too much information could result in a wearying effect: too little information can mean that the campaign is unnoticeable. Generally, good campaigns are long-standing (Atkin 2001), but this also tends to mean that they have large budgets. Much depends on what messages and actions you are trying to promote: however, repetition of messages may be needed over a long term (Tones and Green 2004). An example of the timing of one short-term campaign is provided in case study 5.3.

Planning may also be needed for the long term. The Department of Transport (DfT) (2009c) has an example of their calendar campaigns for the year 2010 available at http://think.dft.gov.uk/think/mediacentre/calendar Note on this calendar that drink driving campaigns are conducted around Christmas, as people are more likely to drink alcohol in the festive season; drug driving campaigns are in the summer (festival time) and at Christmas.

Case study 5.3:   Timing of PSAs in a sexual health campaign

A campaign entitled 'Talk to your kids about sex: everyone else is' (DuRant et al. 2006) used television and radio PSAs alongside billboards and bus advertising.

Four different PSAs of 30 seconds each were aired on three television channels to the 20 counties that had the highest rates of adolescent pregnancy. In each market area each PSA was shown for a week through the day from *Daybreak News* at 5.30 to *Entertainment Tonight* at 8.00 Monday to Friday, resulting in 784 airings of the PSA over a six-month period.

The study found that the frequency that parents reported seeing billboards and television PSAs was associated with frequency parents talked to children about sex-related issues such as contraception. See DuRant et al. (2006) for more information.

CHAPTER REVIEW

This chapter recommends that practitioners consider using more than one source of media – preferably drawn from different categories of media. More successful campaigns use a mass media approach combined with more interpersonal or intrapersonal communication to facilitate discussion and the integration of health issues into the community. This chapter also considers that campaigns should not just transmit messages afresh, but spend some time preparing the target audience for transmission of the main message or event to ensure optimum audience exposure. There may be a number of lessons to learn from the marketing of non-health products in the promotion of health campaigns.

This chapter has:

- identified and explored a range of channels of communication that can be used in campaigns;
- examined the use of experimental marketing, narrative communication, mass media and electronic media in campaigns and considered ways these could be used to reach campaign goals;
- explored ways to utilize different media sources in campaign practice.

FURTHER READING

Corcoran, N (ed.) (2007) *Communicating health: Implications for health promotion.* Sage, London.

Macdowall, W, Bonell, C and Davis, M (2007) *Health promotion practice.* Open University Press, Maidenhead.

Rice, R.E and Atkin, C.K (eds) (2001) *Public communication campaigns, 3rd edition.* Sage, London.

Designing resources

This chapter will explore the steps undertaken in the design of a print-based resource. The steps include planning, message content, readability and suitability, typography, design, interactive features, visuals and a review of the completed resource. As part of the exploration of these steps, other areas covered in this chapter include message framing, fear appeals and brand creation.

This chapter aims to:

- identify the steps in the design of print-based resources
- analyse the role of different design features in the creation of print-based resources
- explore ways to design resources including framing messages, writing styles and adapting content to fit aims
- apply a range of activities to the design of print-based resources

Working in campaigns requires practitioners to engage in the design and delivery of messages in a range of formats. These are usually selected from one of the four media categories highlighted in Chapter 5: audio-visual broadcast; audio-visual non-broadcast; print media; and electronic media. Health practitioners working in the communication field may be involved in the design or re-design of resources in any of these four category areas. Practitioners could find themselves writing press releases and radio advertisements or designing internet pages to reach programme goals. As much campaign work is centred on the best use of resources and the design of the content that will be included in these resources, it is essential that practitioners are able to design (or re-design) appropriate and effective resources.

DESIGNING PRINT-BASED RESOURCES

The steps that should be followed in designing a leaflet are the same as those used in the design of any print-based resource. Most of these steps also apply to materials that are used in other media, such as audio-visual resources. Although this chapter looks specifically at the design of print-based resources, there are also lessons in this chapter for practitioners designing other types of resources such as internet pages or audio-visual resources.

Research indicates that health-related print materials are often unsuitable for the audiences they are designed for. Weintraub et al. (2004) found in prostate cancer campaigns that materials scored poorly in readability, cultural appropriateness and self-efficacy measures. This indicates that the resources examined were less suitable for low literacy and multi-cultural audiences. Similarly, Hoffman and McKenna (2006) found a poor match between reading levels of materials and reading abilities in *stroke* materials, with frequent omission of design characteristics that have been found to improve reader interaction (see section later in this chapter on 'interactive features'). In addition, Kirksey et al. (2004) found that most resources in the pharmacies they examined required reading levels that were too high for the average person to understand.

Research indicates that design features can also be problematic. Harmon et al. (2007) note that poor design and wording of food-related newsletters can mean food-related behaviours are not undertaken. Hall et al. (2008) note that evidence of stereotyping in HPV leaflets may alienate some readers and that most HPV leaflets do not meet the information needs of women. Other problems may relate to the type of messages. For example, a review of HIV/AIDS leaflets from the 1990s suggested that many HIV messages are individualistic in orientation and ignore the wider structural or social factors that impact on HIV (Dodds 2002). It is also important to consider the different characteristics that impact on information retention (Mazor and Billings-Gagliardi 2003). One of the main goals of health communication should be that readers can comprehend and remember the content that is given to them, as inadequate or insufficient information means the likelihood of any attitude or behaviour change lessens (Kools et al. 2006).

When creating print resources, there are a number of key variables to be considered. These can generally be split into eight stages:

1   *Planning*: The target group and stakeholders' identification and the type of resource that will be used, alongside key logistical questions.
2   *Constructing the message*: The aims and objectives of messages, types of message, and content.
3   *Ensuring readability and suitability*: The levels of readability (for example, material reading level) and suitability for the target group.
4   *Using typography*: The styles of type used.
5   *Design*: The organization and structure of content.
6   *Making messages interactive*: Including features that enhance engagement with the materials.
7   *Including visual components*: The images or graphics used.
8   *Review*: The evaluation process at the completion of the resource.

A more detailed analysis of each of these phases is provided below.

Phase 1: Planning

It is important to research the target group (NIH 2008), identify their behaviours, and engage them in the design process. Hoffman and Worrall (2004) also indicate that is it is important to include stakeholders in the design of materials (see Chapter 2 for more information on stakeholders and target group inclusion in the design process). It is also essential to consider in the planning stage what type of resource you want to provide, where it will be distributed and the possible costs such as paper, printing, designers. Print-run numbers (or how many copies you will print) should also be identified. Locations of distribution vary but essentially the location should be where your target group are most likely to be reached. For example, you might consider distributing health information for pregnant women in an antenatal pack or health information aimed at certain minority groups in places of worship such as a church or mosque. Specific information might be tailored to specific locations: for example, information on food labelling might be distributed in a supermarket, or information around harm minimization and illegal drugs in a nightclub. It is possible that you may need permission from the relevant authorities for distribution in some locations and you may need to consider this at this stage. (Chapter 3 contains more information about locations and Chapter 5 has more suggestions on choosing channels of communication.)

Stage 2: Constructing the message

Atkin (2001) suggests there are three basic communication processes involved in campaign messages, namely awareness, instruction, and persuasion. Awareness messages aim to promote awareness or to prompt further information seeking. An example might be a flyer aimed to promote smoking cessation groups in a local area. Instruction messages are those specifying how to do something, for example, teaching a skill or encouraging someone to do something (such as resisting pressure from others to drink alcohol under age). Persuasion messages highlight reasons why a change should take place and are intended to influence attitudes or encourage and strengthen beliefs (for example, promoting the benefits of early screening for oral cancer to prevent cancer. These often utilize theoretical behavioural change models (see Chapter 2). The first decision to make in designing messages should therefore be what sort of message is going to be transmitted; awareness, instruction, persuasion or a combination of these.

Messages should be clear and credible and understood by those with different levels of health literacy, including 'inadequate' or 'marginal' levels (Parker and Gazmararian 2003: 117). Messages therefore need to be clearly identified and stated in the content. This means identifying the aim of the materials and then adapting messages accordingly. Bastian (2008) notes that defining objectives are also necessary for the evaluation of materials, and these should be clearly stated in the plan (Doak et al. 1996).

Designing messages is a complex process. Research by Lillie et al. (2009) noted, for example, that in Kenya, 85 per cent of young people surveyed had heard of ABC in relation to sexual health. This might suggest the effectiveness of the ABC message. However, they also found that only 48 per cent fully comprehended what was meant by A (Abstinence), only 20 per cent B (Being faithful) and 7 per cent C (Consistent condom use). This suggests that a simple ABC message may not be enough without further emphasis on what elements of the message mean.

Activity 6.1:   Matching aims to messages

You are designing a small flyer (A5 size) aimed at parents of children in a secondary school. The flyer aims to encourage them to reduce their speed and drive at 20 mph or below in a newly established speed restricted zone outside the secondary school.

1   What would be your main message(s)?
2   What content would you want to include in your flyer (bearing in mind the small size)?
3   Is your message an awareness, instruction or persuasion message?

Attracting attention

Messages should attract the attention of the audience and engage them in the content of the message. How material is presented on the front of a booklet, leaflet or poster is particularly important, especially as this is the first thing that most people see. Using the target group is important as they will be able to identify features that attract their attention. Not only this, health materials should ensure that they make the behaviour as attractive as possible. For example, Philpott et al. (2006) note that most people have sexual relations for the pursuit of pleasure: sexual health messages should therefore incorporate this such as linking condoms to pleasure. Hoeken et al (2009) consider the use of metaphors in message design. They note that messages based on metaphors may encourage people to think differently about issues and encourage interpersonal discussion. However, the likelihood of misinterpretation is high and practitioners need to be confident that the target audience are clear about message meaning in the planning stage.

Framing the message

Message framing is an important area to consider. Messages can be framed in different ways depending on what the message aims to achieve. Generally messages are defined as gain frame messages or loss frame messages. Gain messages are designed to highlight benefits, loss messages are designed to highlight what you might lose. For example, a 'gain' message might start with the words 'the benefits of turning off your mobile phone while driving …'. A 'loss' message might start with the words 'you could damage your health by using your mobile phone while driving …'. Benefits are translated into a gain frame message, and the damaging effects into a loss frame message.

Activity 6.2: Gain frame and loss frame messages

1 Read the information below and frame one gain frame message and one loss frame message based on the health information about diabetes.

Diabetes Mellitus (type 2 diabetes) may be prevented through modification of a range of lifestyle factors. These include diet and physical activity levels. The reduction of sugar is important, as well as increasing levels of physical activity.

Research findings on whether loss- or gain-framed messages are more effective are somewhat mixed, though there is a tendency for gain frame messages to be more effective (Gerend et al. 2008) and for practitioners to frame messages positively rather than negatively.

Research indicates that other influences may affect whether loss or gain messages prove more appealing. Rothman et al. (1999) propose that message framing may be influenced by different characteristics such as perceived risk. In addition, they suggest that gain frame messages are effective for health-affirming behaviours such as prevention and loss frame messages for illness detection behaviours such as screening. Mann et al. (2004) also propose that different personal characteristics, in this case, approach or avoidance orientation, can impact on message framing. Those with an avoidance orientation responded more to a loss frame message and those with an approach orientation responded more to a gain frame message.

Other researchers propose that time may be important and Tones and Green (2004) suggest that short-term gains might be more effective for young people than long-term gains. Gerend and Cullen (2008) examine the role of both message framing and temporal context (meaning short-term versus long-term consequences) on alcohol use. They found that gain frame messages for short-term consequences of alcohol use were more effective than loss frame messages for alcohol behaviours. For example, those who were exposed to gain frame messages drank less frequently and engaged in less binge drinking. Messages had no effect when they were framed for long-term consequences.

Fear appeal

A fear appeal consists of 'threatening the audience with harmful outcomes from initiating or continuing an unhealthy practice' (Atkin 2001: 61). Although research suggests that the stronger the fear, the more effective the fear appeal message will be (Terblanche-Smit and Terblanche 2009; Witte and Allen 2000), generally fear appeal messages are quite weak. Terblanche-Smit and Terblanche (2009) suggest that groups exposed to low level fear advertising experience low levels of fear and have less positive attitudes to messages when compared to medium and high level fear campaigns.

Some research suggests that fear appeal messages can have a boomerang effect and may be counterproductive (Atkin 2001). For example, being told something is dangerous (such as handling guns or playing with fireworks) can increase curiosity or become a challenge. Chang (2009) notes that in adolescents smoking prevention messages that downplayed psychological benefits increased smokers' favourable views of their smoking, indicating a boomerang effect. Other research considers fear appeals are not recommended for those who are already living in a high fear context, despite strong beliefs from practitioners and target groups that this approach is the most effective (Muthusamy et al. 2009).

There are some best practice guidelines for the use of fear appeal messages. Green and Witte (2006) propose fear appeal messages should be combined with self-efficacy skills, though this can be difficult to achieve through media alone. Advice on how to prevent the 'fear' element from happening is also important in fear appeal messages, so a solution needs to be presented to ensure the person can prevent the behaviour happening, thus decreasing anxiety and increasing behavioural change. One of the best examples of this in the UK is the media campaigns from the Department of Transport (DfT), who for a number of years have integrated fear appeal messages with simple solutions.

Figure 6.1 illustrates a recent campaign example from DfT (2009d). Radio and television adverts are also available with a similar theme at www.dft.gov.uk/think/. The aim of the campaign is to promote the dangers of speeding and encourage

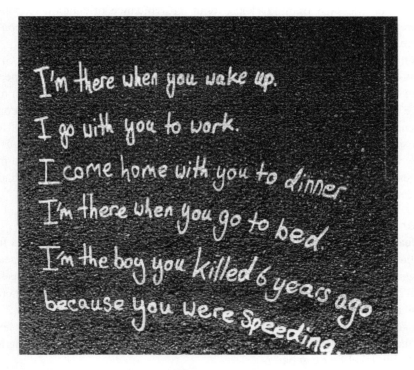

Figure 6.1   Poster from the 'Live with it' road safety campaign
Source: DfT (2009).

people to reduce driving speeds to 30mph. This poster illustrates a fear-raising technique using the idea of being 'haunted' by a boy who was killed 6 years ago. It also provides a simple solution to avoid killing a child; 'drive at 30mph'. An additional example is described in Chapter 8 entitled 'Cow – the film that will stop you texting and driving' (Gwent Police/Tregar Comprehensive School 2009).

If fear appeals are used, caution should be exercised to ensure there are no negative impacts. In the long run, however, fear appeals tend not to be the most effective strategy (Tones and Green 2004) and Atkin (2001) suggests this could be in part because of the limited control we have over messages when they have been received. It is unlikely that fear appeals should make up the sole campaign message strategy. The DfT (Figure 6.1), for example, has a wide range of campaigns and fear appeals only make up a proportion of these.

Use of humour
Humour can be employed for framing messages. However, the use of humour – for example, in the form of jokes, puns or cartoons – does need to be considered very carefully. Not everyone has the same sense of humour, and for some issues that are particularly sensitive, this will not be appropriate. Some authors suggest avoiding the use of humour completely (see, for example, Maslen 2007). This is not to recommend avoiding humour altogether: a light-hearted approach to an issue can be a way of encouraging discussion. Posters by Marie Stopes (2009a), aimed at young people's sexual health, show 'Wilbert', a cartoon penis, wearing a condom in a range of situations with messages such as 'Wilbert and his mates out on the pull' and 'no entry without protection'. You can view these at these links: www.mariestopes.org.uk/documents/Mates.pdf and www.mariestopes. org.uk/documents/Clubbing.pdf

Another example is the Department of Health campaign 'Change4Life' (DH 2009), which uses humour, including cartoon figures, in some of its messages designed to encourage lifestyle change. These are simple health messages with a pun on words or concepts (see Figure 6.2).

The poster in Figure 6.2 contains slogans such as 'it's mind over batter' (instead of the well-used phrase 'mind over matter'), and 'don't veg out, run about!' (with a pun on the words 'vegetable' that you eat and 'vegetate' as in relaxing on the sofa).

Tailoring the message
It is important to consider the characteristics of print information as they affect the retention of information (Mazor and Billings-Gagliardi 2003). There are also differences in acceptability of materials and appropriateness of messages. For example, one target group may prefer leaflets and another booklets. Some messages can be given on flyers, others require more extensive writing.

The style of writing is also important. Mazor and Billings-Gagliardi compared six differently written health materials for stroke. These included short, casual, long and detailed and fictional materials. The fiction group demonstrated the

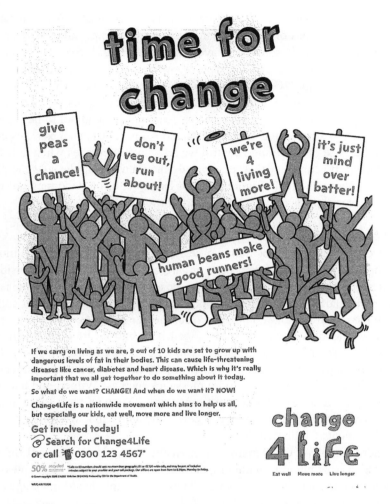

Figure 6.2   Change4Life poster
Source: (DH 2009).

highest 'understandability' of the groups, although there were no differences found in some other variables (such as reading ease). Other authors have found similar findings in relation to story-telling which is also discussed more in Chapter 5.

Complexity of information will tend to exclude readers (Bastian et al. 2003). Content that is specifically tailored for groups with additional needs will require additional work if usual standards do not meet need. For example, you might be working with a group of people who have significant language and health literacy difficulties. Communicating with these groups can be very complicated (Kreps and Sparks 2008). If you want to provide information in different languages, direct translations of leaflets into other languages may not be the most culturally appropriate way to distribute information to your target group. Translations may be inadequate (Larson et al. 2009), and content may not be appropriate, or could be insensitive to cultural norms. It is essential therefore to assess the target groups' needs in the design of culturally appropriate materials, particularly if a translation of language is needed. CDC (1999) indicates that low literacy readers may also interpret information differently from those who are more literate and this may have an impact on the way content is phrased. For example, literal translation of information or poor language fluency may impact on interpretation and comprehension of information. Chapter 4 considers other strategies used in culturally specific materials.

Other target groups may have additional needs that require attention during the design process. Rose et al. (2003) examine the creation of more aphasia-friendly materials, and suggest four principles that can be applied to the design of materials for groups with aphasia. These include using simple words and short sentences, using large, standard font styles, leaving white space, and making use of relevant pictures. Although these principles are similar to other design features, target groups who have additional needs like this may require additional attention in this area, for example, extra large fonts (or other format such as non-print) for those with visual impairments. The assumption should not be that a target group will want different formats (Rose et al. 2003) but this is something that should be explored with a target group.

Activity 6.3:   Cultural relevance of materials

1   Choose one cultural group in the area that you live in who are not the majority population.
2   If you were designing a resource for this group, what other design features might you need to consider in your materials?

Application of theory

Campaign materials should also be informed by theoretical constructs. If a campaign is grounded in a theoretical model, then the model used in resource design will be the same or similar. Even if a resource is stand-alone and not part of a specific campaign, a theoretical model should still inform the basis of the message design. The aim of materials might be to influence attitudes or promote behavioural change. Therefore, the theoretical constructs that can predict successful outcomes are important and should be included to ensure messages match the behaviours or attitudes targeted. Abraham et al. (2007) note that in alcohol education leaflets, the cognitive antecedents associated with alcohol consumption are often not included in alcohol leaflets. This means there is a mismatch between the persuasive techniques that could be used to decrease alcohol consumption and the content in leaflets. Employing the theoretical constructs in the design of materials, as well checking for recommendations in material design for the health topic, is important. Case study 6.1 illustrates the use of the Theory of Planned Behaviour in print-based material design. See Chapter 2 for more information on theoretical models.

Case study 6.1:   TPB and physical activity booklet design

Vallance et al. (2008a) developed a physical activity guidebook for breast cancer survivors based on the Theory of Planned Behaviour (TPB). The elements used were based on previous research and the ten chapters were designed to enhance attitude, subjective norm, perceived behavioural control and implementation intentions. Below are some examples of aspects based on the TPB.

   Chapter 2 of the guide book entitled 'how can exercise benefit me'. The content includes benefits of exercise. Sample content: 'Make it fun. Take up a new hobby that involves exercise …'(p. 178). The TPB variable targeted: *behavioural beliefs*.

   Chapter 5 entitled 'planning for success'. The content includes goal setting (SMART goals). Sample content: 'The next step is to set some exercise goals. Research has shown that setting goals will help you start and maintain your new exercise programme …'(p. 179). The TPB variable targeted: *intentions*.

Stage 3: Ensuring readability and suitability

The 'readability' of a resource refers to the ease or difficulty with which it may be read. The readability of a resource affects its suitability (Vallance et al. 2008b). More attention has been paid to readability of materials than to other design features of materials. The consensus is that materials should be aimed at as low a reading level as possible, preferably below the average reading level for comprehension (Kirksey et al. 2004; Calabro et al. 1996). Studies have found that those who read at a lower reading level comprehend more information than those reading at higher levels, and show more increases in knowledge, attitude and behavioural intention (Calabro et al. 1996). This suggests that it may not just be comprehension that is affected by reading levels of materials, but behaviours too. Average reading levels for the general population in the UK are generally placed around grade 4–6 reading levels which correlate to a reading age of nine to eleven year olds.

   NIH (2008) identifies a number of factors that can increase readability. These include consistency in spellings and definitions, as well as explaining complex terms. Doak et al. (1996) propose some writing guidelines which suggest five main areas to be considered in relation to readability and suitability. These are:

- Write the way you talk.
- Use common words and short sentences.
- Give examples to explain difficult or easily misunderstood words.
- Include interaction (see later section on interactive features).
- Give examples in an active voice, for example, by using 'you'.

Some of these are discussed in more detail below, as are a number of tools that can be applied to written text to assess suitability and readability.

Using common words

Doak et al. (1996) suggest that some common words may be problematic for some target groups. They split these into three types: concept words, category words and value judgement words. Concept words describe an idea, for example, words like 'normal', or 'balanced' or 'healthy'. Category words describe a group of things, for example 'poultry' (meaning chicken, turkey, etc.), or 'exercise' (meaning walking or swimming, etc). Finally, value judgement words describe amounts for action, for example, 'regular', 'heavy', 'moderate'. These can be problematic as they are subject to different interpretations and meanings, for example, 'regular' may mean daily to one person and weekly to another. Where possible it is a good idea to explain words and relay concepts clearly. Instead of writing 'You should eat a balanced healthy diet', it would be better to explain what is meant by 'balanced' and 'healthy'. An alternative would be 'you should try to eat a diet that contains a range of foods, including different fruits (such as apples, bananas and pears), and vegetables (such as carrots, broccoli and tomatoes)'. This way the exact meaning is clearer. See also Activity 6.4.

Activity 6.4:   Concept, category and value judgement words

1   Read the sentences below and identify the concept, category or value judgement words.
2   Revise these sentences to make them clearer for an audience.

- You should drink plenty of water to stay hydrated.
- Apply liberal sunscreen when you are in the sun.
- Wait a while before swimming after you have eaten.

Writing in an active voice and writing the way you talk

Style of writing is an important factor. Writing in the active voice and in a conversational style is recommended (CDC 1999; Doak et al. 1996; Hoffman and Worrall 2004; NIH 2008). In other words, write as you speak, in clear, simple language (Maslen 2007). Writing in a positive way and placing emphasis on benefits if possible (NIH 2008) are also recommended. Terms such as 'you may find' or 'you should try' are better and more encouraging than directive language such as 'you should' or 'you must' (Hoffman and Worrall 2004), which is authoritarian and restrictive in nature. See Activity 6.5 below for more on *message framing*. 　　　　　　　　　　　　　　　 >>

Activity 6.5:   Writing in the active voice and framing messages

It is better to write materials in an active voice, using 'you' instead of terms like 'people' or 'patients'. It is also better to frame messages in a positive way if possible, and use encouraging language. For example, instead of saying 'patients should not

(Continued)

(Continued)

eat saturated fats ...' (passive voice, and negative framing), it is better to say 'you should try and eat less saturated fats ...' (active voice and more positive framing).

1 Have a look at the phrases below and turn the sentences into an 'active' rather than a 'passive' voice.

- Patients should drink plenty of water and rest in the few days after the operation ...
- Don't spend hours at the computer as this can increase postural problems and people can become more susceptible to ...

When writing health materials, it is important not only to be consistent in the use of terminology, but also to use appropriate words and phrases that are neutral, non-biased and not open to misinterpretation. This may require careful consideration of which words to use and how to phrase and depict key points. Health practitioners have a responsibility to ensure materials are correct, appropriate and health promoting (not health damaging). Case study 6.2 gives an example of The Samaritans' (2008) media guidelines to assist the media in reporting suicide in a responsible way.

Case study 6.2:   Appropriate language for reporting suicide and self-harm

The Samaritans (2008) have recognized the role of media in suicide and self-harm and have created a media guide for specific use in the reporting of suicides and self-harm in the media. They note there is some evidence to suggest that use of poor terminology when referring to suicides in the media can lead to glamorizing or sensationalizing suicide and lead to copycat suicides. Alongside a range of information for the media (i.e. dramatic portrayal of suicide in film and reporting tips), they recommend a series of phrases to use when reporting suicide. These include:

Phrases to avoid:	Phrases to use:
A successful suicide attempt	A suicide
Suicide victim	Dies by suicide
Just a cry for help	Person at risk of suicide

Checking readability and suitability

Readability formulas can be applied to health information in order to predict the reading difficulty of printed health information (Friedman and Hoffman-Goetz 2009). Print materials can then be matched to reading levels of audiences. Most readability formulas are quite quick and encourage careful word selection. There are a number of readability formulas that can be used in written materials, both computer and manual based. One of the easiest ways of checking readability if you are designing a resource in Microsoft Word is to do the following:

- Click on 'spelling and grammar' on your toolbar and spell-check and grammar-check your document.
- When the document has been spell-checked and grammar-checked a readability summary may be generated. This summary contains the 'Flesch' readability ease and Flesch-Kincaid grade level.
- For plain English aim for 60 per cent or higher for readability. Grade level 6 (or 6.0) is the equivalent of about age 11 reading level.

All material should be spell-checked and grammar-checked before being piloted with any target groups. Readability does not include visual and design features and it may be difficult to predict readability based on these features (Friedman and Hoffman-Goetz 2007). Instead it is more helpful to consider 'suitability' of materials. The following sections will consider two readability formulas and one suitability assessment that can be used in practice.

SMOG

Manual readability formulas are also available, one of the most common being *SMOG* (Simple measure of gobbledygook) (McLaughlin 1969; 2008). Figure 6.3 illustrates the instructions for using SMOG based on the National Literacy Trust (2009) guidelines who note the age level of reading materials rather than grade level.

SMOG is a simple calculation that can provide a general measure of readability. Practitioners manually count 30 sentences from the materials (10 from the beginning, 10 from the middle and 10 from the end). In these sentences words of three or more syllables are located. Figure 6.4 illustrates the types of words that you would identify in a physical activity resource and how these are broken down into syllables. For electronic text, online SMOG tests are available such as (NIACE 2009) available at www.niace.org.uk/development-research/readability

---

Instructions for SMOG

1. Select three 10 line long extracts of text, one from the beginning, one from the middle and one from the end.
2. Count the number of words which have three or more syllables.
3. Multiply this number by three and circle the number closest to your answer.

1	4	9	16	25	36	49	64	81	100	121	144	169

4. Find the square root of the number you circled.

1	4	9	16	25	36	49	64	81	100	121	144	169
1	2	3	4	5	6	7	8	9	10	11	12	13

5. Add 8 = Readability level.

Most people will understand a readability level under about 10.

Figure 6.3 Guidelines for using SMOG

Source: Adapted from National Literacy Trust guidelines (2009).

Number of syllables	Number of syllables	Words broken into syllables
One (not counted in SMOG)	sport	sport
Two (not counted in SMOG)	active skiing	ac-tive ski-ing
Three	exercise cycling	ex-er-cise cy-cle-ing
Four	education activity	ed-u-ca-tion ac-tiv-i-ty
Five	orienteering	o-ri-en-teer-ing

Figure 6.4   Identifying and counting syllables

Activity 6.6:   SMOG grading of a health resource

1   Find a health booklet or leaflet with at least 30 lines of text. Calculate the SMOG grade reading level using the instructions in Figure 6.3.

SAM and suitability formulas

SAM (Suitability assessment of materials) is a useful, widely used tool for evaluating print materials (Vallance et al. 2008b). It has 22 items grouped under six headings including content, literacy demand, graphics, layout/typography, learning stimulation/motivation, and cultural appropriateness. Raw scores are calculated and turned into a percentage that is then used to assess suitability on the following scale: 70–100 per cent superior, 40–69 per cent adequate, and 0–39 per cent not adequate. Although suitability formulas are mostly used for paper-based resources, they may also be applicable to IT-based resources such as internet pages. As the SAM requires an individual judgement on a number of items, it is also a good idea to have more than one person assessing the suitability of the resource. See p. 119 for where you can access this resource.

Stage 4: Using typography

The general consensus is that font size 12 or larger is appropriate for written resources. Research by Harmon et al. (2007) found that readers of newsletters preferred larger fonts even when this meant less information could be included. Hoffman and McKenna (2006) note a font size of at least 12 should be used, and research by Eyles et al. (2003) suggest font size 14. Research on internet-based materials suggests that Arial, Courier and Verdana are the most legible with Comic Sans the least (SURL 2002).

Serifs are the structural points on a letter that lead the eye on to the next letters. They work well in written print-based resources and are the most common font used in resources such as books, magazines and newspapers. Sans-serif fonts are those without the bars on the letters and are more likely to be used in short text. For online resources Verdana is often seen as the most readable font. It is a broad and spacious font and leaves clear square space for each letter (Scratchmedia 2009). Arial is also preferred on computer-based resources. Sans-serif fonts are recommended for online resources due to factors such as screen resolution and font sizes.

Italics and capital letters are hard to read, especially in whole sentences (Doak et al. 1996; NIH 2008). Bold font can be used to highlight key points. Thus font size 12 or above is recommended, with possible preferences on style of font used suggested by the target group. Finally, some colour content can be difficult to read (CDC 1999) and these tend to be light colours on darker backgrounds (rather than dark colours on light backgrounds). It is therefore better to use dark inks, rather than light ones, and to avoid ink colours like yellows that can be difficult to see. Ideally black on white or dark blue on cream or white are optimum for writing (Maslen 2007).

Stage 5: Design

A number of design features can help to increase reader interaction and the comprehension of resources. In a booklet, for example, a contents page is helpful, as well as placing content in a logical order. Hoffman and McKenna (2006) found that subheadings are frequently omitted from print resources, even though they can aid understanding and are cited by a number of authors as important in the design of materials (for example, Doak et al. 1996; Maslen 2007). Organizing information using sub-headings may be a good way to present information. It is also logical to have larger headings at the top of the page with sub-headings getting progressively smaller.

Larson et al. (2009) found that question-and-answer and true/false formats were preferred. Bullet points and simple question and answer formats are also easier to understand as they are usually structured for lower reading levels, for example, shorter sentences, and indicate to the reader where to look for the information they want.

Attractiveness of a resource is also important, although there are trends (concerning colours and design) that can change over time (Bull et al. 2001). Colour and design can enhance attractiveness if features can be linked to a specific audience known to be attracted by certain things such as children liking cartoons. Even the type of paper used has been found to be important in the design of resources. Springston and Champion (2004) found that colour was important in the adaptation of a brochure for African Americans on mammography screening. Pastel colours were originally proposed by the designers, but the target group indicated that these were European, rather than African, colours. The target group proposed colours such as red, green, black and gold which were more African, as well as the inclusion of the Kente cloth design (a Ghanaian 'cloth of kings' print) that has deep historical roots. The inclusion of the Kente cloth design was seen to be associated with respect and reinforced the fact that the brochure was specifically designed for the target group.

Stage 6: Making messages interactive

Hoffman and McKenna (2006) note that features encouraging reader interaction are often absent from resources. Doak et al. (1996) suggest such techniques as goal setting, short question and answer (Q and A), circling the correct answer, or selecting between true and false could be used. Personal touches can include spaces for names on booklets (Doak et al. 1996), which are particularly important for patient information booklets, or those with a personal meaning. For example, if you were turning part of a leaflet on sun safety into a more interactive format, you could try writing quiz questions such as 'What time of day should you seek shade?' Alternatively you could turn content into True/False propositions, for example, 'You should seek shade in the hottest part of the day between midday to 3.00pm' True or False? Another example is to leave space for goal setting. For example, you could have a tear-out sticker that says 'next time I go to the beach these are the sun safety things I will take with me' and leave a space for a list. Gallivan et al. (2007) in their diabetes brochures allowed readers to write three reasons for controlling their diabetes, three things they would do in the next three months to improve diabetes control, and three people who could help them with their action plan.

Activity 6.7:   Turning content into interactive content

You have written the following content as part of a leaflet to promote safety in a factory where heavy machinery is often operated on the warehouse floor.

> There are a number of hazards in the job that you do. These include injuries from incorrect operation of machinery. You should receive yearly training on the machines that you work on, alongside first aid training and manual handling training. Please make sure you are up to date with your training. Accidents are also more likely to happen if you are operating machinery when you are tired, unwell or you have been drinking alcohol or taking medication.

1   Read the content and try to formulate two quiz questions that you could write instead of the text.
2   Write a true/false question that could be used.
3   Taking into account the fact that workers need to be yearly trained, what could you write that might encourage goal setting in this resource?

Stage 7: Including visual components

Visual components can help to reinforce printed messages and engage the reader (Kulukuluani et al. 2008). There are a variety of ways that visuals can be used in printed materials. Houts et al. (2006) propose four uses of images. These are:

- to draw attention to the material and the message;
- to help people comprehend the information;
- to increase recall of messages;
- to increase the likelihood that people will adhere to a message.

These authors also indicate that simple drawings are more effective, perhaps because they minimize distractions. For example, if you use photographs, the camera catches a variety of other detail. Cultural relevance is also important in image use, as some images can be interpreted in different ways (Houts et al. 2006). The general consensus is that, if the visual image does not add something important to the understanding of the material, then it should not be included (NIH 2008). Therefore it is helpful to include images (for example, a picture of the heart or bowel) if they enhance understanding of conditions connected to these pictures.

Concise captions for pictures (Houts et al. 2006; NIH 2008; Hoffman and Worrall 2004) may be used to aid understanding and interpretation of images. A list of practice recommendations has been proposed by Houts et al. (2006) in the use of images in health materials. These include ensuring pictures support key points, linking pictures and content together to guide interpretations of pictures, and using images that are culturally sensitive. Using simple pictures is also desirable.

Images and pictures can help to engage readers, for example, cartoons such as those associated with the QUIT smoking campaign (QUIT 2007) (see Figure 6.5). The person in this cartoon has covered themselves in NRT (Nicotine Replacement Therapy) patches. The cartoon caption 'don't overdo it' helps to lighten the mood of stopping smoking and promotes the idea that NRT, although helpful for quitting, should be used as recommended (i.e. using one patch). There may also be some benefits to using cartoons with younger children as a way to engage them. The Department for Transport (DfT 2009e) uses cartoon animation for its child road safety advertisements available at http://talesoftheroad. direct.gov.uk/

As with humour, the use of images requires careful consideration to ensure that no groups are alienated, stigmatized or offended. For example, research by Dodds (2002) highlights one Asian-focused HIV leaflet with an image of a cartoon Asian doctor pictured wagging their finger throughout the leaflet. This serves to promote the role of authority and alienate those Asian groups who do not associate sexual health with medical doctors.

Stage 8: Review

Materials should be pre-tested (NIH 2008). Evidence-based information is important, and should be up to date and non-biased, as well as informing and empowering readers (Bastian 2008). It is also helpful to check for comprehension, attractiveness, acceptability and engagement in the materials (CDC 1999) to ensure that your target group will accept the materials.

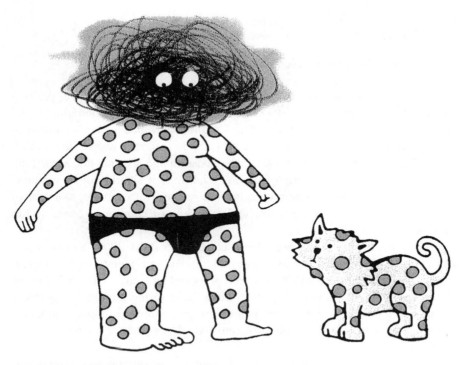

Figure 6.5   QUIT (2007) 'Don't overdo it'
Source: Poster reproduced with kind permission of QUIT (2007).

BEST PRACTICE IN THE DESIGN OF RESOURCES

A number of authors have provided recommendations for designing effective materials (see for example CDC 1999; Doak et al. 1996; Hoffman and Worrall 2004; McKenna and Scott 2007). These can be applied to any print-based resource. Table 6.1 summarizes key points from the literature concerning the design of print-based resources. These are divided into eight summary sections of pre-planning, message content, readability and suitability, typography, design, interactive features, visuals and review (as was the content of the literature above).

Activity 6.8:   Designing a leaflet using best practice

1 Using the summary of recommendations in Table 6.1 to help you, work though each of the eight stages discussed in this book and develop an outline for the leaflet below.

> The topic of your leaflet is: To increase awareness of the hazards in the home associated with childhood accidents under five.
>
> The target group is parents and carers of young children in one ethnic minority group (choose one group).

Table 6.1 Summary of recommendations in the design of print-based resources

Pre-planning	• Involve stakeholders and target group • Identify the type of resource i.e. poster, leaflet • Identify the locations where the material will be distributed
Message content	• Identify the main aim • Determine key information needed to achieve aim • Identify the main messages • Limit the number of messages, i.e. 2–3 maximum • Link main messages to a theoretical model • Consider the content format i.e. Q&A • Ensure content is culturally sensitive • Tell readers what they should do and what they gain
Readability and suitability	• Aim for a low grade reading level i.e. 6th grade. • Use short sentences and short words • Write in the active voice, i.e. 'you' • Test materials using a readability formula
Typography	• Use font size 12 minimum • Avoid using italics and CAPITAL letters • Use a dark colour ink • Use **bold** for key points only
Design	• Organize topics logically • Leave plenty of white space • Use sub-headings, bullet points, simple Q&A or cues i.e. arrows • Sequence information with important information first • Use appropriate colours, i.e. dark ink on light background
Interactive features	• Add features to increase interaction, i.e. quizzes, blank spaces to write, goal setting or diary pages
Visuals	• Only use an image if it increases understanding • Choose images that match the text • Use simple line drawings • Place images in context, i.e. parts of the body • Add captions to all images • Ensure images are culturally relevant • Use good quality images • Choose colours that appeal to the specific audience
Review	• Content should be accurate, evidence-based, non-biased, culturally appropriate and referenced • Post test for comprehension, attractiveness, acceptability, engagement with material

ADDITIONAL IDEAS

Using ideas from other disciplines

It may be possible to utilize ideas and good practice from other disciplines to assist in the design of health-related resources. Maslen (2007) notes in a book on copywriting that showy writing and long-windedness do not work. He suggests that keeping focused on the reader, being concise, using story telling, asking questions, and being creative are all helpful in the area of marketing. The book also recommends using a list of contents, page numbers, colour coding, putting keywords inside stars or arrows. Although these principles have not been formulateded specifically to a health setting, they remain strategies that ensure the reader is guided through a written document and can assist in the understanding and readability of a document. There are also a number of advertising companies who utilize billboards, posters, bus wraps and other channels to promote a range of products. Their work is available for viewing on websites which can help to give ideas to practitioners in the health field. Two examples include CBS (2009a) Inspire me gallery at www.cbsoutdoor.co.uk/Inspire-me/Gallery/ and JC Decaux (2009) campaign gallery available at www.jcdecaux.co.uk/campaigngallery/

Creating a brand

An additional element to a campaign may be the creation of a brand. This can strengthen the relationship between consumers and producers and can help to add value to objects (Evans et al. 2008). Branded health messages are commonly theory-based (Evans et al. 2008). Good campaigns will consistently use the same style of resources, such as similar colours and messages. This could be classed as branding information. For example, the use of logos on materials ensures consistency and is a symbolic representation that helps to differentiate products from each other (Evans 2008). Levy et al. (2007) in their campaign 'It ain't Brain Surgery' which aimed to reduce traumatic brain injury (TBI) in skiers and snowboarders used the campaign slogan and logo on posters, brochures and stickers for helmets. Atkin (2001) suggests that continuity devices such as logos, slogans, jingles and messages are all important to increase campaign memorability.

CHAPTER REVIEW

This chapter has recommended a series of steps to follow when designing print-based resources. This includes an eight-stage design process which allows practitioners to design or re-design effective and appropriate resources for campaigns. This chapter has also considered the application of readability and suitability tools.

This chapter has:

- identified the steps in the design of print-based resources and considered the best practical recommendations for using these design features in the design and creation of a resource;
- explored ways that resources can include design features such as loss or gain framing messages, using different writing styles, and adapting content to fit aims;
- identified the use of readability and suitability tools and considered ways to increase the effectiveness of resources using these techniques.

FURTHER READING

Centers for Disease Control and Prevention (CDC) (1999) *Scientific and technical information: simply put, 2nd edition*. CDC, Atlanta, Georgia.

Doak, C C, Doak, L C and Root, J H (1996) *Teaching patients with low literacy skills, 2nd edition*, Lippincott Company, Philadelphia. Available at www.hsph.harvard.edu/healthliteracy/doak.html.

Hoffman, T and Worrall, L (2004) Designing effective written health education materials: Considerations for health professionals, *Disability and Rehabilitation* 26 (19) 1166–1173.

For more information and assessment sheets for SAM (Suitability of Assessment materials) see either the Doak et al. (1996) or CDC (1999) sources above.

Evaluation in practice

Evaluation has long been recognized as an important part of campaign design and implementation. It can be a difficult element to incorporate into campaigns. This chapter seeks to identify the main challenges involved in the evaluation of campaigns and examines practical ways to overcome these. This chapter also considers the role of a five-stage process of evaluation in campaigns – the stages comprising formative, process, impact, and outcome evaluation, plus feedback. We also examine alternative strategies and activities that could be included in the evaluation process.

This chapter aims to:

- identify challenges to evaluation and consider strategies to overcome these in practice
- describe a five-stage process of evaluation and apply these steps to campaign practice
- identify activities that can be used in evaluation strategies to ensure effective evaluation

EVALUATING CAMPAIGNS

'Evaluation is the systematic application of research procedures to understand the conceptualization, design, implementation and utility of interventions' (Valente 2001: 106). Evaluation is essential for demonstrating values and credibility of campaigns (Suggs 2006) and also provides a contribution to the evidence base on campaigns. Evaluation is also used to help improve effectiveness, engage with audiences, respond to change and allocate resources (The Communications Network 2008).

Evaluation is essential at all stages of a campaign. Its scope includes the delivery of a campaign, the materials that are used, the aims and objectives and planned outcomes. Evaluation is generally conducted to find out what worked and to help plan for future activities. Evaluation should therefore be integral throughout a communication campaign, rather than an 'add on' at the end. Evaluation is a process that continues over time (Wellings and Macdowall 2006), rather than simply being used at a single point in time. It may be thought of as a circular process, rather than a linear one.

Evaluation is not a rigid process consisting of a pre-defined list of questions to be answered. Whilst it is clear that some questions, such as those concerning the comprehensibility and understanding of a message, are important to all campaigns, other questions will be campaign-specific. Factors such as number of visitors to a website or number of people booking a free screening test, for example, will only be suitable if the campaign includes these elements. The evaluation methodology need therefore to be flexible and one that 'respects [the campaign] character and the way they work' (Wellings and Macdowall 2006: 158).

CHALLENGES OF EVALUATION

The importance of evaluation is now widely accepted. However, evaluation is often not done well. A number of common difficulties occur frequently. These include trying to evaluate your own work objectively (Wiggins et al. 2007) and also budget and time constraints. Another difficulty is knowing what to measure. This may result in practitioners measuring everything (which is very time- and resource-consuming and often impractical) or, on the other hand, not measuring enough things.

Coffman (2002) suggests in campaigns there are a number of challenges to evaluation. Four of these in particular warrant further attention below. These are:

* horizontal and vertical complexity;
* unpredictability;
* wider context of the campaign;
* the lack of a control group.

Horizontal and vertical complexity relates to the aims of a campaign. Often campaigns seek to produce outcomes at three different levels: (1) environmental change such as agenda setting; (2) community changes such as changing norms; and (3) individual change such as behaviour change. This makes evaluation challenging.

Even when campaigns are carefully planned, there will inevitably be an element of unpredictability. This could consist of the wider media context, for example, you may launch a campaign at the same time that other news stories are released that compete against your campaign. Alternatively, there may be a misinterpretation of your message by the media or by the general public. It is also difficult to determine who has seen your messages, and which aspects they respond to. Not all unpredictability is entirely negative, for example, though a record number of users to a website may cause the website to crash or telephone help lines to become blocked, it is good to have so many visitors to the site!

The wider context of a campaign refers to the environment beyond the campaign. It can be extraordinarily difficult to separate out a campaign message from other messages that are transmitted and received at the same time. For example, an evaluation of a message about safe nightclub drug use to 16–20-year-olds will need to take into account messages given by nightclubs, bars, friends, family, schools, police or other influential sources. It may be difficult to isolate the effects of one message from other messages and causal claims need to be clearly substantiated with evidence.

Finding a control or comparison group can be difficult. Most research standards dictate that the gold standard in research is a randomized control trial (RCT), meaning that there is a carefully identified control group who do not receive an intervention. Because most communication campaigns are broad in scope, it can be difficult to identify a group to use as a control that has not been exposed to the campaign in some way. For example, billboard, bus wraps or posters in one town could be seen by anyone visiting, working or commuting to that town even if they do not live there.

Activity 7.1:   Identifying challenges to evaluation

You have been working on a campaign to encourage university students to actively commute (for example, by walking or cycling) to and from a university campus in a large city in the autumn semester. At the same time the local council has been encouraging residents of some boroughs to leave their cars at home to reduce congestion and pollution on the roads and has opened a number of new cycle lanes in the city.

1   What challenges might you face in evaluating your campaign?
2   How might you overcome these?

OVERCOMING THE CHALLENGES

No campaign exists in a vacuum and recognition of the backdrop to a campaign is essential. Wider environmental, media, social and political factors all have an impact on communication. Wellings and Macdowall (2006) refer to this as 'background noise' as it indicates that a range of other 'noises' are competing for the target group's interest. Background noise concerns not just the wider environment such as where a target group lives: it combines with interpersonal factors such as peer pressure or parental influence. Distinguishing just what influences who and when can be almost impossible, although behaviour change theoretical models can assist to some extent (see Chapter 2). There are a number of strategies that a practitioner can use to help ensure that evaluation findings are attributable to specific campaigns.

Practitioners should ensure that their messages are able to compete with other messages. A black and white, badly written, and poorly photocopied flyer cannot hope to compete with a well-designed campaign. A campaign needs well-produced, clear and memorable messages and these are what you will want to evaluate in your process and impact evaluations and they will also need to be pre-tested with the target group (formative evaluation). You may want to consider 'branding' your programme (see Chapter 6): then recall questions can also be asked about the campaign brand. Keeping a media clippings file is important (as discussed below) as is documenting what other events are taking place on a wider scale during your campaign, such as political events. Finally, consideration of a control group or time series component is also good practice – again, this is discussed further below.

Formative and impact evaluation should lessen the likelihood of something unpredictable occurring. If elements of the programme, such as budget and resources, are measured throughout, this can ensure the campaign stays on track. In addition, close monitoring of the message effects (recall, responsiveness or behavioural changes) can ensure that the message has the desired outcome.

One element that practitioners need to consider in the evaluation of campaigns rests in the recognition that campaigns that heavily rely on mass media are in essence 'mass' in nature and effect size of messages is going to be small. Synder (2001) proposes that generally mass media campaigns have size effect of around 5 per cent. Thus aiming for 50 per cent of the population changing their behaviour is unrealistic. Campaign goals need to be grounded in realistic outcomes.

A control community strengthens the evidence base for evaluation. However, establishing a control group can be difficult in campaigns due to their broad nature. Most research would recommend a pre-post evaluation design where a group is measured before the intervention and after the intervention. In some studies this is possible. For example, a sun safety programme in the USA and Canada in ski resorts was able to gather baseline data and pre- and post-test data over a period of time so as to measure campaign effects (see Andersen et al. 2009). This built on previous research where control groups from different ski resorts in similar locations were available. Similar communities of 'inside' settings may be possible, for example, comparing two similar schools or two GP surveys. This will require care to eliminate contamination of the control, as children visiting the control school or people accessing services offered by different GP practices will be able to access campaign messages thus biasing the control group.

Activity 7.2:   Establishing a baseline or control group

You are working with a travel agent company on a campaign to increase the personal safety of 18–30-year-olds in certain holiday resorts in one country in Europe. This includes distributing a free safety pack with samples of sunscreen, a money belt, condoms, and a 'what to do in an emergency' advice booklet to all 18–30s booking with the travel agent. In addition talks by the travel representatives will be given, focusing on keeping oneself safe.

1   Who could you use as a control group?
2   How would you establish a base line measurement?

An alternative suggested by Bauman et al. (2006) is the use of a time series component as a comparison measure. This means that the same group is measured at different time points, such as three times before and three times after a campaign. Essentially this means measuring a group's knowledge, attitude, behaviour or other variables before the campaign has occurred and then measuring again the same variables over different time points after the campaign. This might be 3 months, 2 months and 1 month before the campaign, and then 1 month, 2 months and 3 months after the campaign. This does not replace the notion of a control group, but does allow the practitioner to establish a comparison in the absence of an available control group.

It is important that everyone working on a campaign agrees on evaluation methods before evaluation takes place. Shared decision-making for evaluation is important. A study by Adams et al. (2009) in New Zealand found that different funders had different expectations as to what would be measured. The Ministry for Health wanted formative and impact/outcome evaluation that included surveys on social relation of place. The Department for Child, Youth and Family were interested in the process evaluation of organizational and decision-making processes and the community was initially suspicious of proposals where they could not see the value of these in the project. It will be difficult for an effective evaluation to take place unless there is a shared understanding between the main groups involved. Deciding what to evaluate can be a complex task and McKenzie et al. (2005) note that finance, participants, validity, access to resources such as computer software will also be important in deciding what to evaluate.

FIVE STAGES OF EVALUATION

Evaluation of communication generally consists of four stages, namely (1) formative; (2) process; (3) impact; and (4) outcome evaluation. In addition a fifth variable of feedback can also be incorporated into this. Other writers in the area of health communication suggest similar stages (see, for example, Bauman et al. 2006). Formative evaluation is pre-evaluation of the main materials and strategies

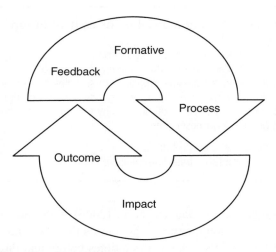

Figure 7.1   Five-stage evaluation cycle

of a campaign before the campaign commences (Chapter 3 has more information on formative research processes). Process evaluation is an evaluation of the implementation of the campaign process and looks to measure the programme progress. Impact evaluation is the immediate effects of the campaign. Outcome evaluation is the more long-term effects of the campaign. Feedback is the distribution of the campaign's findings back into the evidence base. Figure 7.1 illustrates these stages in a circular format, although generally campaign work starts with formative research.

Formative evaluation

Bauman et al. (2006) propose that formative evaluation is the most critical step in developing campaigns. This is generally the stage where the campaign material and strategies are evaluated before (and sometimes during) the campaign. It may be a time of pre-testing messages and resources and designing and developing concepts. Gallivan et al. (2007) undertook ten focus groups with people with diabetes in different cities in America to learn more about their target group and to pre-test concepts, scripts and themes. The campaign theme line 'Control your diabetes. For life' came from the focus group discussions reflecting the target group's desire to take care of their own diabetes and enjoy better quality of life.

All campaign materials and resources need to be pre-tested. This includes checking instructions, proofreading booklets, and testing telephone lines and web-links. Atkin and Freimuth (2001) suggest five elements to measure in pre-testing messages, namely attention value, comprehensibility, relevance, strengths/ weaknesses, sensitive or controversial elements. These five elements can be applied to all media-based resources and this process should be undertaken in conjunction with the target group. Table 7.1 later in this chapter summarizes a list of possible questions to ask in the formative evaluation phase.

Establishing a baseline measurement

If you want to measure a change, you will need to establish a baseline figure and this is usually done at the formative evaluation stage. This can be a simple list that has informed your campaign messages, for example, myths about pregnancy in a group of adolescents. Alternatively it can be a measure of knowledge, attitude or behaviour based on a survey or pre-questionnaire. Whatever measure is chosen, it should be closely linked to what the campaign wants to achieve. For example, a campaign promoting recognition of iron deficiency in children might start by measuring how many people recognize two signs of iron deficiency. Alternatively the campaign might be linked to behaviour. For example, a campaign to increase the number of people buying and serving children vegetables that have a high iron content might start by identifying shopping and cooking habits.

Activity 7.3: Using formative evaluation

You are working on a print-based campaign to increase the number of school children under 11 in three schools wearing protective helmets when using bicycles. You have designed an activity booklet and free helmet stickers for the children and a parents' information leaflet.

1   What questions could you ask if you were conducting a formative evaluation of this campaign? (Just think about formative evaluation.)
2   What methods would you use to collect your data? (Chapter 3 might also give you some ideas for this.)

Case study 7.1:   Back pain advertisements

Barker et al. (2007) carried out a study to examine back pain information in the mass media. They found a broad acceptance of mass media message, especially television. NHS sources were deemed acceptable, credible and reliable but government sources were viewed with scepticism. In addition, they noted comments on a range of advertisements. Advertisements with the word 'work' in were seen as more negative as they advocated a return to work which was linked to unsympathetic employers. In addition, terminology such as 'gentle exercise' and its meaning were seen as conflicting in the media. It is suggested that the meaning and acceptability of mass media messages should be explored prior to the implementation of a campaign.

Process evaluation

Process evaluation should lead to campaign improvements and support programme objectives. It helps practitioners to determine why a programme is successful or not (Saunders et al. 2005). Process evaluation has recently received more attention in the literature. It generally refers to an evaluation of the implementation phase of the campaign and the documentation and analysis of the way the campaign works.

Different researchers suggest attempting process evaluation in different ways. Saunders et al. (2005) suggest six steps which include describing the programme, acceptability, resources and contexts. Other areas for process evaluation include distribution, placement and exposure of messages. Distribution looks at what the campaign distributed, how, when, where and how many. Placement concerns where paid and unpaid coverage is generated. Exposure concerns where the target audience sees the campaign. DuRant et al. (2006) suggest asking about the number of times the campaign was seen, whether the audience remember the message, and how convincing the message was. In addition, variables such as the number of people who can recall the brand or the name of the campaign and other such measures may be useful. Questions therefore might include:

- reach of the messages
- interpretation of messages
- receivership of messages
- location(s) of messages
- exposure levels of messages
- number of times messages are received
- problems and challenges of delivery.

In addition, process evaluation may include meetings, observations, surveys or interviews with project staff, stakeholders, the target group or other interested parties. Campaigns can also have steering groups and process evaluation feedback often consists of feedback to steering groups. Hooker et al. (2009) describe a study to promote more walkable neighbourhoods for seniors. The process evaluation required from programme leaders included lessons learned, specific accomplishments, challenges and barriers and changes in policies. They also included elements such as 'what would others need to know if they were doing something similar?' Table 7.1 summarizes a list of possible questions to ask in the process evaluation stage.

Roe and Roe (2004) propose that dialogue boxes may be a useful tool for process evaluation. These are essentially evaluation forms with the question 'Is there anything you would like to say to ...' and then a list of options such as campaign staff or the technical team. The comments are then collated into one form and distributed at the next meeting. They note that dialogue boxes can help to demystify the evaluation process and take away the notion that evaluation is 'done' to people. They also note that they allow people to express something on paper and equalize power as no-one knows who wrote what. They do suggest establishing some group rules for elements such as appropriate and inappropriate content.

One of the main reasons for process evaluation is the identification of barriers that hinder campaign progress. If these can be identified and responded to accordingly in the process evaluation, then the campaign is more likely to be successful. Problems include lack of resources, conflict, epidemics, broken equipment, and so on and these need to be carefully monitored.

Table 7.1   Examples of questions to ask in each stage of the evaluation process

Type of evaluation	Examples of variables to evaluation	Five examples of questions to ask in different campaigns
Formative	Comprehensibility Relevance Sensitivity Suitability Understanding Clarity Attractiveness Appeal	Is the material attractive? Do the target group understand the messages? Are the messages clear? Are all the materials spell checked? Does the message appeal to the target group?
Process	Recall Service use Number of times aired Number distributed Barriers to campaign development	Is everything going according to plan? Does the target audience understand the message? Is the target audience able to recall the message? How many leaflets have been distributed? How many times has the radio advertisement been aired?
Impact	Access Recall Change to attitude Change to behaviour Change to beliefs Change to values Change to psychological variable Number of preventive behaviour achieved	Have people accessed the stop smoking service helpline service? Are people able to recall the road safety message correctly? Have beliefs about the benefits of fruit and vegetables increased? Are more people accessing the local swimming pool? How many recycling bins have been distributed?
Outcome	Change to behaviour Mortality increase/decrease Morbidity increase/decrease Environmental change Policy change Political change	Has there been a decrease in the number of people reporting theft? Has there been a reduction in CHD from sedentary lifestyles? Has there been an increase in screening for testicular cancer? Has there been a change to local tobacco smoking policies? Are there more streetlights in the main street?

Activity 7.4:   Using process evaluation

You are evaluating a walking group that a leisure centre has set up and has been promoting in the local community. At the start of the campaign the leisure centre distributed door-to-door flyers in the local area, posters in community locations (such as bus stops and community notice boards) and maps for walkers to follow of routes in the local area. A number of local walkers have been attending each week, although this has decreased over time.

1   What questions could you ask if you were conducting a process evaluation of this campaign?
2   What methods would you use to collect your data? (Chapter 3 might also give you some ideas for this.)

Case study 7.2:   Promoting hand hygiene in hospitals

Thomas et al. (2005) undertook a campaign to increase hand hygiene behaviours in five hospital wards. Although the impact of these posters was measured through elements such as observation, the posters themselves were also an important part of the campaign. The first posters were evaluated through focus groups and the findings of these informed the development of consecutive posters. The team found that posters had a positive influence on hand hygiene but the lack of human qualities in images in early posters (for example, those showing germs) was flagged up. This enabled the campaign to move away from images of cells and germs and develop images based on focus group findings of the more human images of people washing their hands. This illustrates how involving the target group in process evaluation might be helpful for message design as the target group can re-design or adapt messages to increase their effectiveness, thus promoting engagement in the campaign process.

Impact evaluation

Impact evaluation measures a campaign's immediate effectiveness, for example, short-term changes such as changes to behaviour or in service use. It is conducted on immediate conclusion of the campaign. Evans et al. (2009) suggest that practitioners need to be clear whether it is the efficacy of messages or another aspect of the campaign which leads to effectiveness, such as the audience reaction. They suggest that we need more efficacy studies that look at message effects. This suggests impact evaluation may focus on the efficacy of the intervention, and the immediate impact that messages may have had on the target group, such as immediate recall or recognition of a brand.

Table 7.1 summarizes a list of possible questions to ask in the impact evaluation stage.

Activity 7.5:   Using impact evaluation

You are evaluating a prostate cancer campaign that has been running in a large bank. The campaign used email to send prostate cancer information to all males in the organization. The email included a description of prostate cancer, prostate cancer statistics and a link to a national website for further information. The website was designed predominantly in a question and answer format with scenarios, case studies and links to further information which include a helpline number. Around 1000 emails were sent to male members of staff. Website traffic figures indicate around 250 more hits a day to the website than the usual website traffic in the first week the email was sent. The most popular page visited was 'how to recognize the signs of prostate cancer'.

1   What questions could you ask if you were conducting an impact evaluation of this campaign?
2   What methods would you use to collect your data? (Chapter 3 might also give you some ideas for this.)

Case study 7.3: Measuring exposure and awareness in the 'Checkpoint Strikeforce' campaign

Checkpoint Strike force (Beck 2009) was a campaign in Maryland, USA, that responded to an increase in alcohol-related traffic fatalities. Roadside sobriety checkpoints were used alongside paid and earned media (local news items) to promote the campaign. A number of measures were used in the evaluation of this campaign and these included measuring exposure and awareness of the campaign.

Exposure was measured by questions such as: *'In the past 30 days have you personally gone through a checkpoint where police were looking for impaired drivers?'* If respondents said 'Yes' they were labelled 'exposed'. If respondents said 'No, to all these questions, they were labelled 'unexposed'.

Awareness was measured by questions including: *'In the past 30 days have you seen or heard anything about a checkpoint where police were looking for impaired drivers?'* If respondents said 'Yes', they were labelled 'aware'. If respondents said 'No' to this question, they were labelled 'unaware'.

For more information, see Beck (2009).

Outcome evaluation

This step refers to the main health outcomes, such as the reduction of mobility or mortality. It is an evaluation that takes place after a period of time has elapsed in the campaign. The time may be divided into different periods. For example, a stop smoking programme may measure at 6 weeks, 6 months and 12 months. Or a campaign to encourage pregnant women with low iron levels to increase their iron intake during their pregnancy and the early weeks post-birth might follow up these women when their babies have reached six months. The evaluation may also look at wider measures such as policy change.

Table 7.1 provides a list of possible questions to ask in the outcome evaluation stage.

Activity 7.6: Using outcome evaluation

You are evaluating a campaign that aims to increase parental skills and coping strategies in young teenage parents and parents-to-be under-18 presenting at a local health centre. The campaign includes an antenatal pack of resources aimed at younger people and an invitation to an under-18s mother and fathers group (NP group). The NP group teaches new parent skills for eight weeks including bathing a new baby, breastfeeding, safety in the home and coping skills. The antenatal pack has been distributed to around 60 new parents and parents-to-be under 18 over a six-month period. Two NP groups have run over consecutive eight week periods. Attendance at the NP group has been high with around 40 mothers or fathers attending at least four sessions.

1 What questions could you ask if you were conducting an outcome evaluation of this campaign at 6 months?
2 What methods would you use to collect your data? (Chapter 3 might also give you some ideas for this.)

Case study 7.4: Measuring recall, beliefs, intentions and behaviours

Berry et al. (2009) undertook a mixed methods evaluation of television advertisements targeted at older adults that promoted fruit and vegetables and physical activity. They used a population level telephone survey and focus groups. The survey examined recall, beliefs, intentions and behaviours.

An example of a question to measure beliefs was:

'For me eating a healthy diet will reduce my chances of getting serious health problems' (Responses were rated 1=not important to 5=very important).

An example of a question to measure intentions was:

'How likely is it that you will eat the recommended number of fruit and vegetables over the next month (Responses were scored on 0–100 per cent on an 11 point scale).

For further information, see Berry et al. (2009).

QUESTIONS TO ASK IN THE EVALUATION CYCLE

Table 7.1 on p. 129 lists sample questions that could be asked during the formative, process, impact, or outcome stages of evaluation. These include questions connected to the content discussed under each sub-heading of the evaluation cycle. This is not an exhaustive list of questions but rather a list of examples to encourage practitioners to consider their evaluations of their own campaigns.

Feedback

The final stage of the evaluation cycle consists of feedback. This element is often neglected in campaigns, which is disappointing because future campaigns need to build on the evidence created from good practice. Even if campaigns have not been very successful, other practitioners will benefit from knowing the outcomes of these campaigns for their own work. There is a strong recommendation that results should be disseminated and a plan for how this will take place can be agreed in the planning stages of the campaign. Valente (2001) suggests five ways of dissemination of evaluation results, namely (1) scheduled meetings; (2) conferences; (3) reports; (4) online; and (5) academic journal papers. A report is the standard format.

It is important to disseminate good practice to stakeholders, communities, academics, politicians or other interested parties. When you are deciding how to disseminate your findings you will need to think clearly about time frames and need-to-know data. If you are seeking to publish in an academic journal, then note there can be a considerable time delay before the results are published.

Activity 7.7: Dissemination of findings

You have been working on a HIV prevention pilot programme with construction workers in a number of towns in Southern Africa. You have some encouraging findings from your campaign that aimed to promote condom use in this group and reduce rates of HIV transmission.

1 Who might want to know about these results?
2 How would you feedback your results to them?
3 Where could you publish your findings relatively easily and quickly?

COST-BASED EVALUATION

Not all communication campaigns use the five-step evaluation model described above. Some interventions may just use particular elements of it. Others may use economic or cost effective evaluation. Measuring the relative cost of a campaign means you calculate the relative financial cost. For example, a cost effective analysis would include costs of the programme and also its benefits, expressed in quantifiable terms such as the number of life years gained. A cost utility analysis examines the values attached to health gain such as the use of QALYs (Quality Adjusted Life Years). Research by Solberg et al. (2008) looked at the health impact and cost effectiveness of alcohol misuse reduction interventions in primary care through a systematic literature review. They examined variables such as: the costs of screening, including both patient and physician time, per capita expenditure on annual societal costs of alcohol abuse, cost savings from screening and counselling, the medical costs of alcohol attributable disease and the cost of alcohol-related crime. There are some problems concerning this type of evaluation. Cost input is generally more straight forward as it will include less quantifiable elements such as materials, people, or resources cost. However calculating cost output can be more difficult as you have to attach values to variables like quality of life. McKenzie et al. (2005) provide more detailed information on cost-based evaluation.

EVALUATION TECHNIQUES

There are a number of ways in which data can be collected for formative, process, impact and outcomes evaluation. The Communications Network (2008) has identified a number of common evaluation techniques. They include interviews, focus groups, surveys (on-line/in person), observation, content analysis and quantitative data collection and analysis. Some of these are described in more detail in Chapter 3. When selecting your data collection technique, there are a number of variables to consider. These include the target group, what is being evaluated and current skills. These are discussed in more detail below.

First, careful consideration should be given to which methods the target group is familiar with and able to participate in. In the USA, Sun et al. (2007) collected evaluation data for a breast cancer practices campaign amongst Chinese women through interviews in locations that the women frequent. Locations included day care centres, garment factories, churches, grocery stores, English as a second language classes and the streets of Chinatown. Interviews were conducted in English, Cantonese or Mandarin (two Chinese languages).

Mitchell and Branigan (2000) note that other characteristics of the target group requiring consideration include:

- Are they homogeneous (alike) or heterogeneous (mixed)?
- Are they a natural group or will they need to be brought together for the task?
- Are they experts or lay people?
- Will they be easy to recruit?

Although these were noted in relation to using focus groups, these questions can be applied to all target groups. For example, part of the outcome evaluation might be to conduct 15-minute interviews with working parents in a supermarket in the evening. Given that most people have been working in the day and may be rushing through an evening shopping trip, this may not be an attractive prospect unless incentives are provided or the benefits of participation are highlighted.

Second, the question of what is actually being evaluated is important, for example, attitudes, beliefs, values or the impact, exposure or reach of a message. Different data collection techniques suit different purposes. Focus groups may be a good way of examining group perceptions such as attractiveness of a resource or understanding of a message, but they are not very good for gaining individual opinions, evaluating knowledge or tracking behaviour change.

Third, time, budget and resources are also important. Face-to-face interviews are a good way of gaining in-depth knowledge, but they are also time- and resource-consuming. In addition, developing resources such as a questionnaire and analysing the results accurately can be time-consuming and labour-intensive. Finally, the skills of the evaluator are important. Designing a questionnaire, interview schedule or conducting a focus group may require skills that evaluators do not have.

Generally, it is recommended that a mixture of quantitative and qualitative methods is used. Not all data collection requires the participation of the target group. For example, collecting figures from attendance at classes, changes to healthcare access locally, the number of operations performed or other similar measures may be useful. Chapter 3 gives some more ideas of ways to collect data that do not require the target group's assistance.

Activity 7.8:   Evaluation techniques

You want to evaluate a campaign that has been running in a local clinic to promote 'active aging' in older people. The campaign aimed to increase the amount of physical activity that clients attending the local clinic were undertaking each week. All of the older people have fallen at least once, and are at risk of further falls which is why they were originally referred to the clinic. They have been given a range of exercises to do at home, as well as encouraged to increase their daily physical activity levels.

1   What sort of evaluation questions might you need for process, impact and outcome evaluation?
2   What methods could you use to collect data?
3   Where would the data collection take place and with whom?

MONITORING

All campaigns should as a matter of course keep track of activities (1) within the campaign (such as the placement of messages), and (2) outside the campaign (newspaper or radio coverage). Although the actual behavioural or knowledge impact of a campaign cannot be evaluated through monitoring, aspects such as scope and coverage are covered (WRAP 2006). A selection of elements that are important to the campaign are needed. WRAP (2006) has some examples, but standard questions include:

- the type of media and where and when it appeared and what it was, for example, coverage in a news column;
- the main topics covered, for example, the main issues or themes;
- the size of the article, for example, column length and lines;
- the visual impact, for example, photographs or layout;
- the prominence of the article, for example, was the campaign mentioned at the top of the article?

To locate the news items, Gould et al. (2004) suggest using a newspaper database such as Lexis-Nexis (which requires a fee, although it is available in most public and academic libraries). It is available at www.LexisNexis.co.uk or a free online newspaper database such as 'googlenews' http://news.google.co.uk/. Alternatively, locating the most popular newspapers and searching these by hand or online is possible. In the UK the highest broadsheet newspaper circulations are those for *The Daily Telegraph* (www.telegraph.co.uk). *The Times* (www.timesonline.co.uk) and *The Guardian* (www.guardian) (NRS 2009). The tabloid with the greatest reach in the UK is *The Sun* (www.thesun.co.uk) (NRS 2009). There are also a number of news channels such as BBC News available at http://news.bbc.co.uk/.

Activity 7.9:   Monitoring a health issue in the news

1   Choose one health issue that interests you and make a list of search terms that you might use to look for a news item on your topic.
2   Log on to the internet and access google news using http://news.google.co.uk/
3   Search the news items for the last week and select one article of news about your health issue.
4   Answer the following questions based on the five questions in monitoring activities section:

    (a)   What type of media have you found, what is the name of the newspaper?
    (b)   What are the main topics covered?
    (c)   How many written lines long is the article?
    (d)   Is it visually attractive, for example, photographs or layout?
    (e)   How prominent is your health issue in this news item?

5   Are there any other questions that you could ask about the news item that could be useful for your analysis?

MEASURES OF REACH

One measure that can be used to assist with evaluation data collection is the media impression of a campaign. Though these figures may not be accurate, they do give some idea of the scope that the campaign can reach. There are a number of standard ways of measuring 'opportunities to see' (OTS) (essentially the number of people who have the opportunity to see an article in the media, on a billboard, on a bus or train, and so on). Each country will have its own means of capturing and providing this data. In the UK, sources include:

- National Readership survey – Reach of magazines and newspapers available at www.nrs.co.uk;
- Postar – Billboard and other outdoor advertising which provides links to other advertising agencies www.postar.co.uk;
- CBS Outdoor – Bus and tube advertising www.cbsoutdoor.co.uk;
- RAJAR – Listener numbers for radio (generic rather than specific to advertising) www.rajar.co.uk.

Each organization has their own way of evaluating the effectiveness and figures of reach of their advertising. For example, Postar measures travel patterns and also estimates vehicle and pedestrian traffic at individual places and eye contact and visibility.

MEDIA ANALYSIS

Media analysis is a good indicator of the changes in the social context (Wellings and Macdowall 2006: 160) surrounding a campaign. An analysis can be undertaken to help practitioners understand how key health issues are represented and to check the other health media messages that are transmitted at the same time as campaign messages. These can be quite complex to undertake and Gould et al. (2004) explains this process in much more detail. Essentially, a media analysis looks at articles from a set time frame (for example, six months) and uses appropriate search terms to locate articles. Key search terms need to be agreed first and then these are entered in the date restricted news databases (Lexis-Nexis or Google News). A manageable number is between 100 to 200 papers, so they may need first to be hand-sifted down, or search terms may need refining if a high number of articles are located. A series of questions can then be applied to each article. See Table 7.2 for a list of common subheadings used in a media analysis. These include generic information such as dates and locations of information, who presents the story, and how the health issue is presented.

Table 7.2   Common subheadings used for media analysis

Subheading	Explanation of sub-heading
Type	Articles can be classified into types such as opinion, news, fictional, review or feature
Placement	Location of where the story is noted, for example, where in the paper (front, middle, back) and the name of the paper
Timing	Date and time of the story
Topic	Examination of how the issue is presented. This could be prominence such as the main issue, or a sub-section of the story
Spokesperson analysis	Consider who is telling the story or being quoted
Framing analysis	This is partly if the issue is a positive appeal or negative appeal (see Chapter 6 for more on message framing). It may also be how the issue is presented such as the genre of the story (fact, statistical, humour, sympathetic, first person narrative or other category)

EVALUATING ONLINE COMMUNICATION

Given the move towards information technology in communication campaigns, the chance that some campaign elements will be electronic is quite high. These electronic elements include the use of the internet, *blogs* and social networking sites (Chapter 5 discusses a range of these in more detail). As campaigns seek to compete in a media-crowded world, these sites may well become more widely used in health communication. Evaluation of information technology is not well represented in the literature, but essentially the main components of the five-step evaluation cycle already discussed also apply to evaluating electronic media. The fundamental difference will be the different types of elements evaluated.

Peattie (2007) proposes four 'C's that should be considered in the evaluation and development of websites. These are:

- Community – such as message boards, blogs, *chat rooms* that help build support
- Content – the extent of relevant up-to-date information and interaction such as quizzes
- Commerce – the merchandise available
- Connectivity – the ability to connect to users on the site as well as the authors though mechanisms such as feedback or polls.

Electronic media provides a number of benefits to evaluation that are not available from general audio-visual media. On internet sites this includes the use of web-site counters that count the traffic visiting the site and page histories that count who visited which pages. In addition, there are a number of features that can be created on internet sites or other social networking sites that could be used in evaluation. These include:

- number of questions asked in an 'Ask a question' section;
- number and type of discussion strands, or topics created in discussion;
- number of messages or emails posted;
- number of people joining a group or cause;
- number of people downloading a screensaver, game or other application;
- number of people voting on a topic (for example 'should vaccines be compulsory – yes or no?');
- number of people creating a profile page, virtual person or other personal indicator.

On the Diabetes UK (2009) website, visitors to the website can undertake a short 2-minute test giving them instant feedback on their diabetes risk. This data would be able to provide you with the number of people who visit the site, who are at risk of diabetes and a idea of the demography of the visitors to the site (such as age, ethnicity, sex). You can view the 2-minute test at www.diabetes.org.uk/measure%2Dup/

Activity 7.10:   Evaluating a website

1   Have a look at this website: www.condomessentialwear.co.uk
2   List all the features on this website that promote engagement with the website content.
3   What features could you use in an evaluation of this website?

UNCONVENTIONAL EVALUATION METHODS

Some means of evaluation may be specific to particular campaigns. For example, group activities or tasks may be used as an evaluation alongside the use of drama or role-play as participants put into practice what they have learnt. Ritchie et al. (2007) used the medium of story as a way to undertake process evaluation of a smoking cessation group. They saw this as having the advantage of being able to contextualize local culture and different influences on smoking.

If a campaign was looking at improving skills (such as the ability to perform first aid), then it is logical to evaluate the campaign by checking whether it can actually perform the task. If a campaign has been looking at increasing positive attitudes toward young people with a physical disability in a school setting, the target group could be asked to incorporate these messages into a play or role-play at the end of the campaign. These methods may also be important if target groups are not proficient in English or are not able to express themselves well verbally. Writing songs, dance, music, poems, plays or stories could all be included as part of the evaluation strategy.

Activity 7.11:   Unconventional evaluation

You are evaluating a campaign that aimed to encourage young people aged 13–17 in an inner city area to stop carrying dangerous weapons (knives and guns) on local streets.

1   What unconventional ways of evaluating could you ask this group to do during (process evaluation) or at the end (impact or outcome evaluation) of the campaign?

CHAPTER REVIEW

This chapter has considered the role of a five-stage evaluation cycle. It recommends that practitioners incorporate these elements of evaluation into their campaigns at the conception level of the campaign. A number of suggestions have been given for questions to ask at each stage, including when to use electronic media, and practitioners are encouraged to consider these questions alongside formulating some of their own for their campaign-based work.

This chapter has:

- identified a five-stage evaluation cycle of formative, process, impact, outcome and feedback for campaigns;
- examined difficulties associated with evaluation of campaigns and suggested ways to overcome these;
- considered additional ways to incorporate evaluation measures into practice including monitoring activities, media analysis and unconventional ways of evaluating.

FURTHER READING

Coffman, J (2002) *Public communication campaign evaluation: An environmental scan of challenges, criticisms, practice and opportunities*. Harvard Family Research Project, Cambridge, MA.

Thorogood, M and Coombes, Y (eds) (2000) *Evaluating health promotion*. Oxford University Press, Oxford.

8

Overview: ten campaigns

This textbook has presented a range of theoretical examples and creative ideas to apply to the planning, design, and implementation of health campaigns. Readers should now be in a position to commence planning, designing and implementing health campaigns by following each chapter and its suggested guidance.

The guidance provided above can be summarized in the following ten recommendations for practice:

1. Use a planning model to guide campaign design and development.
2. Set SMART aims and objectives that are consistent with methodology.
3. Identify an appropriate behavioural change theoretical model to inform campaign design.
4. Spend time collecting data from the target group to assist in the identification of target groups, health issues and settings.
5. Identify the target groups' key influential characteristics and variables and include these in the campaign design.
6. Use multiple media and appropriate channels of communication.
7. Ensure adequate and appropriate exposure to campaigns.
8. Use channels of communication that help to promote interpersonal discussion.
9. Follow the eight-step planning model for designing new resources or re-designing old ones.
10. Use a model of evaluation that incorporates process, impact, and outcome evaluation methodology.

If health campaigns follow these ten recommendations, they are likely to result in more effective, appropriate and creative campaign designs that meet the aims of public health and health promotion practice.

To illustrate the contents of this book in practice, ten campaigns will be explored. They use a variety of those methods outlined in this textbook to achieve their aims. It is hoped that these suggestions might encourage practitioners to explore some of these campaigns in more detail and consider the possibilities of applying not only the ten recommendations for practice above, but also the use of additional techniques to their own areas of practice.

This chapter is not designed to discuss the *best* ten campaigns. Rather, it highlights ten recent campaigns that utilize different methods and means of disseminating their main messages and which are grounded in a selection of the ten recommendations highlighted at the start of this chapter. They have been selected for their variety in terms of size, health topics, and target audiences. It is hoped that, by exploring these campaigns and following the suggested website links, practitioners will be able to see the theoretical recommendations provided by this book come alive in practical contexts.

1. VERB™

VERB™ was a social marketing campaign run by the CDC in the USA (CDC 2009). The campaign ran from 2002–2006. Its findings are now available in a special edition of the *American Journal of Preventive Medicine* 2008, 34 (6) 'The VERB™ Campaign Not About Health, All About Fun: Marketing Physical Activity to Children'. The focus of VERB was on marketing physical activity to 'tweens' in order to increase and maintain physical activity among tweens (youth aged 9–13) and to encourage them in breaking rules, changing games, and having fun. The campaign combined paid advertising, marketing strategies, and partnership efforts to reach the distinct audiences of tweens as well as targetting parents and influential others such as teachers. Advertisements were tailored to general market audiences as well as specific groups such as African American, Asian American, and Hispanic/Latino.

Information on the different channels used (for example, TV, radio, print), the types of activities and events as well as a wide range of resources are available at www.cdc.gov/youthcampaign/advertising/index.htm

2. CHANGE4LIFE

The DH campaign 'Change4Life' (DH 2009) uses animation to promote lifestyle changes in physical activity and healthy eating. The campaign uses multiple media sources that contain the same animated figures to promote a selection of messages. On the website visitors can join other families in making lifestyle changes and undertake a five-minute questionnaire in return for which they are offered free personalized action plan, view tips, holiday ideas and can enter a postcode to find local activities. When joining the campaign you are issued with a kit that contains stickers, booklets and other materials to encourage a lifestyle change. The campaign also uses a variety of advertising means such as television, billboard and bus stop advertising.

View the website at:
www.nhs.uk/change4life
View the advertisements at www.youtube.com/view_play_list?gl=GB&hl=
en-GB&p=00CDFCE1A6996B45
Read more from the Department of Health about this campaign at www.dh.gov.
uk/en/News/Currentcampaigns/Change4Life/index.htm

3. CONDOMS ESSENTIAL WEAR

Condoms essential wear (2009) aims to normalize condom use amongst sexually
active 18–34 adults. The main message is that condoms are 'essential' wear to
protect against STIs. The website contains a range of resources. This includes a
section (called 'get your facts right') addressing myths and information to
increase knowledge in sections all about protection and infection. There is also
an interactive quiz, 'How much do you know?'. Interpersonal communication is
encouraged through 'spread the word' where visitors to the site create a 'Private
Dick porn film' to spread the word about condoms. The site is also linked to a
free confidential hotline and you can also find a local clinic by entering a postcode. The site also features incentives in a 'special offer' section which encourages visitors to regularly visit the website.

View the website at www.condomessentialwear.co.uk

4. 2 MINUTES

The 2 Minutes British Heart Foundation campaign encouraged people to tune in to
'watch your own heart attack' as 'the most important two minutes you'll ever see'
(BHF 2009). The 2-minute TV event screened once on national television on 10
August 2008 starred Stephen Berkoff and was designed to illustrate what it feels
like to experience a heart attack and encourage recognition of the signs of a heart
attack. Celebrity-driven short 'teaser' advertisements on the TV and radio together
with online and outdoor advertising were used to promote the event. The video is
also available on the 2-minute website and is available in media such as YouTube.
The website also encourages sharing of the video by signing once you have
watched the video and encouraging people to 'spread the word' by sending the link
to others. Evaluation statistics by Thinkbox (2008) found that over 6 million people
tuned into this event, the website has attracted over 350,000 unique website visits,
and the film has been viewed on YouTube over 61,000 times. Knowledge and
awareness levels of symptoms of a heart attack have also increased.

View the short film and the website at www.2minutes.org.uk/
Find more about the campaign strategies and evaluation from www.thinkbox.tv/
server/show/ConCaseStudy.1395

5. COW – THE FILM THAT WILL STOP YOU TEXTING AND DRIVING

Gwent Police and Tredegar Comprehensive School (Wales) made a short PSA film to reduce SMS texting on mobile phones while driving. The film was made with a budget of £10,000 with a local film producer (Peter Watkins-Hughes). The PSA was launched on YouTube and claims not only local interest but global interest especially in the USA.

View this PSA at www.youtube.com/watch?v=KF0_7qC6YFo. Please note that this video shows disturbing and graphic images.
More information about the campaign can also be found at www.gwent.police.uk

6. DROP THE WEAPONS

A number of London Metropolitan Police campaigns have centred on gun- and knife-related crime and incidents in recent years. The recent campaign sees the creation of a website www.droptheweapons.org/ (Trident 2009b). This website contains songs and lyrics, film and artwork and viewers can upload their own videos centred on guns and knives. The website contains a range of testimonals from gang members who have been involved with guns and knives and been sent to prison. You can view these at www.droptheweapons.org/gallery.html.

One feature of the website is a 'Choose a Different Ending' film. This is an interactive video which allows visitors to decide what happens next. It is aimed at 13–15-year-old male Londoners. Viewers interact with the film and choose what to do and decide how it all ends. In 'Choose a Different Ending', viewers 'decide whether to live or die'. The campaign aims to dispel the myth that carrying a knife gives you protection and encourages young people to think carefully about their decisions by showing them the consequences of carrying a knife: death, shame on their families or prison.

Advertising of this film is through online sites, MTV channels and other media channels accessed by this target group.

View 'A Different Ending' at www.youtube.com/adifferentending
Read more about the London Metropolitan Police knife and gun campaigns at www.met.police.uk/campaigns/anti_knife_crime/index.htm

7. YOOBOT

The British Heart Foundation (2009) has created a website where school children are encouraged to make their own avatar in the form of a Yoobot. Children are encouraged to create their own Yoobot, add their own face by uploading a photograph and then experiment with the future of their Yoobot. Children feed their Yoobot whatever food they like and they can travel through time to see what the Yoobot looks like when it is old. It has been developed to encourage children to think more about their food.

View the Yoobot website at www.yoobot.co.uk/

8. DRUG DRIVING: YOUR EYES WILL GIVE YOU AWAY

Drug driving campaigns by the Department of Transport (DfT) are usually concentrated around the Christmas and summer periods (DFT 2009c). 'Drug driving: your eyes will give you away' was launched at the end of the summer 2009. Materials include a television advert, posters, screen savers, leaflets and resources for festival based campaigns. Figure 5.1 illustrates the festival 'glasses' given away at festival events. The main messages include that your eyes will give you away (that you have been taking drugs) and that the penalties are the same for drink driving; a fine, a ban and a criminal record. The website includes an alternative journey planner and answers to questions such as 'can police spot a drug driver?'. You can also add the website to social networking pages.

The Department of Transport is responsible for a range of campaigns each year connected with road safety. Some of the more recent ones include 'Moment of doubt' (drink driving) and 'Live with it' (speeding).

For more information on the drug driving campaign see www.dft.gov.uk/think/drugdrive/
View the resources at www.dft.gov.uk/think/drugdrive/mediacentre.shtml

9. TIME TO CHANGE

Time to change (2009) is a large-scale campaign aimed at ending mental health discrimination. The campaign is run by a number of organizations and uses a number of strategies including mass participation events, education, community projects, challenging policy and law and changing the way people view mental health via mass media. The media campaign materials include radio, TV, outdoor and washroom door advertisements. In the summer of 2009 two short films were released and advertised on websites such as popular newspaper websites. The films rely on viewers' fear and stereotypes and attempt to challenge these alongside emphasizing the role of family and friends in mental health.

View the films at www.time-to-change.org.uk/online-films
View the TV, radio and press advertisements at www.time-to-change.org.uk/what-were-doing/our-campaign/about-campaign/tv-ad
Read more about the campaign at
www.time-to-change.org.uk/home/

10. MOVEMBER

The Prostate Cancer Charity (2009) runs a campaign called 'Movember'. This is a worldwide campaign that started in Australia. The campaign aims to increase awareness of prostate cancer in men through a charity event that runs every November. Men start the month clean shaven and join the cause as 'Mo Bros' when they grow a moustache over the month of November and raise money and awareness of prostate cancer. Essentially the campaign aims to make men's health a fun issue and encourage interpersonal discussion about prostate cancer.

Read more about the international campaign at www.movember.com/ and the UK campaign at http://uk.movember.com/

Activity discussions

This section contains discussions for the activities that are found in each chapter of this book. These are not designed to be definitive answers to each activity but as suggested examples to the activities.

CHAPTER 1

Activity 1.1: Unplanned outcomes

1   Positive effects could include weight loss, reduction in fat, eating healthier foods, being more aware of dietary intake, increased self-esteem or more positive body image. Negative effects could include stress or anxiety due to negative body image, low self-esteem, dramatic dietary changes or behaviours leading to eating disorders.

Activity 1.2: Stages in the planning process

1   Planning stages for a campaign could include a range of factors. Essentially these should have included most of the steps in the nine-point planning model: rationale, needs and priorities, aims and objectives, selection of theoretical model, method, resources, budget, evaluation, action plan, implementation and feedback.

Activity 1.3: Planning using the nine-step model

There are a number of ways this campaign could have been designed. Some examples are below.

1   The aim is to increase the number of parents who brush their children's teeth correctly for three minutes at least once a day. A theoretical model could be: the Theory of Planned Behaviour (for the role of subjective norm i.e. parental influence). The method: an oral heath pack i.e. with a parent's leaflet. Design: This describes the design of the method. i.e. the Sticker will say 'My teeth are as clean as croc's' with a picture of a crocodile, or the leaflet identifies three reasons why parents should brush their children's teeth. Resources: This will be a list of resources and how you have spent the £1000 budget, i.e. £500 for 500 toothbrushes. Action plan: This will be a plan of who undertakes what and when from the start to the end of the campaign. Implementation: This would be when the campaign is undertaken. Feedback: This would say when you feed back, to whom, and how.

Activity 1.4: Designing campaigns using the 4 Ps

Product is physical activity

Price is the cost of physical activity and the time spent on other things such as groups, homework and socializing.

Place is the location you want to use to promote physical activity, i.e. in the school playground or in a local park.

Promotion is the ways you will promote your small fold-out booklet.

Activity 1.5: What factors are important in Stage 3?

1 Examples include poor sitting or standing position, inappropriate footwear, working above recommended hours before having a break, poor seating or current health levels of cashiers.
2 Examples include messages that centre on correct posture and positioning at checkouts or knowing your working rights (taking a break).

Activity 1.6: Methods, strategies and materials

One method would be to promote physical activity at a low intensity such as walking (to address uncomfortable), that is free such as a local park (to address cost and access).

Method: Walking in a local park on planned routes.
Strategy: Identify circular walking routes in the local park that take an easily followed route i.e. flat ground. There will be five walks between 15 to 30 minutes long to encourage progression to 30 minutes with seated places for rest. Maps will be distributed by district nurses on their visits to leg ulcer patients who are able to walk for more than 15 minutes unaided and can easily access a park via foot, private or public transport.
Materials: These include a short leaflet on benefits of walking in the local park specifically for leg ulcer patients, park plan, paper, cardboard, computer, coloured inks and laminating equipment.

CHAPTER 2

Activity 2.1: Formulating different objectives

1 Possible objectives could be:
   To increase parental knowledge of three possible triggers of a child's asthma attack.
   To encourage parents to smoke cigarettes outside of the house to retain a smoke-free household.
   To ensure parents are able to make the link between their smoking behaviour and their children's asthma.

Activity 2.2: Matching objectives to your aim

1 Examples include 'To ensure every ward has fully stocked supplies of hand gel over a six month period' or 'To increase the number of people who are able to suggest one reason why keeping hands clean is important by 50 per cent.'

Activity 2.3: Which methods best suit which objectives?

1 (i) Behavioural.
2 (i) Knowledge.
   (ii) Mass media such as posters, or interactive classroom activities.
       Methods could include asking children to draw pictures of things you do before you wash your hands and using these for posters.
   (ii) Stories, radio or drama, workshops, mass media, one-to-one or small group.
       Methods could include designing an audio story around older people and diabetes diagnosis.

Activity 2.4: Choosing stakeholders

1 (i) Supermarket owners, supermarket managers, supermarket in-store staff, food manufacturers, shoppers, local residents, local and national diet related charities i.e. BHF, local GP surgery staff, health promotion\public health department, healthy eating programmes in local area.
   (ii) Factory owners, young 16–20 factory workers, other factory workers, factory floor managers, local sexual health (GU) clinics, local GP surgery staff, local and national sexual health charities or organizations, parents, influential others, i.e. church leaders, condom manufacturers.

Activity 2.5: Using the HBM in practice

1 Example messages include: The earlier you identify breast cancer the easier it is to treat, so you can still be around for your family when they need you.
   You are important to your family, this means you need to take care of yourself. Early screening for breast cancer is vital.
2 In church-based locations i.e. community rooms, or family-based activities locations, i.e. local parks.

Activity 2.6: Targeting variables

1 Attitudes (for example, acceptability of assault in public), general social influences (for example, most people important to you think a boy can assault a girl), outcomes expectancy (for example, partner would become more angry if I prevent him/her from assaulting you).
2 Messages could centre on violence being socially unacceptable, they could highlight the consequences of assault for both the assaulter and the assaulted, and promote mutual respect in relationships, i.e. hitting or punching is not acceptable in a relationship.

Activity 2.7: Matching what your target group say to theory

1 Perceived Behavioural Control, the Theory of Planned Behaviour.
2 Perceived susceptibility/severity, the Health Belief Model.
3 Attitude, the Theory of Planned Behaviour or Precontemplation, the Transtheoretical Model.
4 Subjective norm, the Theory of Planned Behaviour.

CHAPTER 3

Activity 3.1: Prioritizing health issues

1 This answer will be different depending on your own country.
2 Your rated importance of this, morbidity, mortality, your location, and the current issues in your country will influence which came first.

3   It is likely these will be different by developed or developing countries, as health issues differ in importance. For example, in the UK, HIV mortality and morbidity are low, but deaths from cancers are high, and generally safe drinking water and road infrastructures are in place.

4   Aside from current and feasible solutions to the problem, data might be collected on areas such as morbidity and mortality figures such as hospital admissions, disability registers, years of life lost (DALYs) or impact of the solution.

Activity 3.2: Designing questions to assist campaign focus

An example based on the Health Belief Model.

1   Possible questions include: How susceptible do you see yourself to suffering from ill health as a direct result of your diabetes? If you got sick as a direct impact of your diabetes, how severe do you think this would be? What are the benefits to losing weight? What barriers do you experience to taking physical activity?

2   A different theoretical model would collect data on different questions and would choose different variables to focus on.

Activity 3.3: Choosing a setting for road safety messages

1   A pub or bar.

2   Example answers include: Those who drink alcohol access this location. Drinking alcohol takes place here. Additional unhealthy behaviours may include smoking. Alcohol may have an impact on judgements. Bar memorabilia i.e. bar mats, t-shirts, flags, glasses, soft drinks promotions and posters, leaflets, radio or video clips in washrooms or main bar could be used. Influences of peers and alcohol may skew judgement.

3   This example may still use this location, but you could integrate other locations outside of the pub/bar too.

Activity 3.4: HPV (Human papillomavirus) vaccine promotion in a community setting

1   Need to meet with community leaders and gatekeepers especially men and highlight the importance of HPV in female health.

2   Key decision-makers in the community including males and females.

3   Community locations that both men and women access, for example, universities, community centres or places of worship.

4   Messages should be culturally sensitive and seek to correct public confusion as well as promoting benefits. They should also be addressed to men as well as women and include the benefits of HPV vaccination and why it is important to women in a family context.

Activity 3.5: Source validity and reliability

1   Possible appropriate sources include journal articles, published documents from government, organizations, charities, institutes or health services.

2   An example is NICE (2008) mental well-being of older people available at: http://guidance.nice.org.uk/PH16 answers will differ for this question depending on the source used.

Activity 3.6: Including the excluded

1 Access non-traditional settings such as barbers, coffee houses or beauty salons.
2 Non-traditional methods, for example, stories, drama, pictures, photographs, songs or competitions.

CHAPTER 4

Activity 4.1: Health information sources based on age

1 Friends, younger family members, radio, television, health professionals, groups or clubs.
2 Family, friends, magazines, internet, schools or television.
3 Friends, magazines, groups or clubs, television, radio, internet, location specific i.e. pubs, clubs, bars.

Activity 4.2: Campaigns for men and women

1 Messages aimed at women will emphasize group support and friendship. For example, 'Make new friends and join a new walking group for people like you.' Messages aimed at men will emphasize new skills and knowledge. For example, 'Join the local gym and learn how to control your diabetes through new exercises.'
2 Possibly. If you are emphasizing different messages and different activities and men and women are unlikely to participate together then you may have two campaigns, or a 'brother and sister' campaign under one umbrella.

Activity 4.3: Variables that influence diet

1 In the UK there are a diverse range of ethnic groups. For example, African groups may eat vegetables such as yams or plantain which many white groups do not.
2 Examples include culture and acculturation, location to shops or markets that sell foods, cooking skills.
3 One example is promoting fruit and vegetables that are culturally specific in images and leaflets aimed at different groups.

Activity 4.4: Five cultural strategies

1 Peripheral, evidential and linguistic strategies are generally cheaper to use as they require adaptation of existing materials although they may be less effective than strategies that involve target groups more. Constituent involving and sociocultural strategies engage the target group more and may be more effective, but may require more time and financial costs.
2 Depending on finance and time, it is likely that the last two strategies (constituent involving and sociocultural) will have a bigger impact on the target group due to their involvement in the campaign design.
3 Yes. The higher strategies involve less time and contact with the target group than the lower strategies.

Activity 4.5: Targeting physical activity to religion

1 Messages could be linked to messages in faith, sermons or scripture. For example: 'Be healthy in faith and body'.

Activity 4.6: Tailoring to philosophies

1   Messages could be centred on caring for the environment or encouraging physical activity in open environments such as in parks: 'actively commuting to work helps reduce pollution'.

Activity 4.7: Attitudes, beliefs and values

Examples include:

1   Positive attitude to consuming high fat foods, belief that these foods taste nice.
2   May have mixed attitudes towards foods depending on the links he makes between weight, heart condition and high fat foods. Belief that high fat foods may be linked to weight, places high value on the nice taste of foods like chicken and chips.
3   May have a positive attitude to looking after his health due to his diabetes, believes that high fat foods are to be eaten in moderation and places low value on these.

Activity 4.8: Beliefs and methods

1   Messages are likely to be linked to fertility and infertility and may include notions of perceived susceptibility. An example message might be 'Infertility is not as common as you think, don't take the risk and use condoms every time.'

Activity 4.9: Identifying and defining a target group

1   This could be any target group of your choice, for example 18-year-old black Caribbean men, or 60-year-old white women with grandchildren. Make sure you have converted all of the questions on the checklist.
2   The response to this would depend on your answer but psychological factors and behaviours are more likely to be harder to answer than social factors.
3   You would need to research your target group thoroughly using a variety of methods, for example internet or media research, alongside meeting or observing your target group.

Activity 4.10: Tailoring information in practice

Examples could all be centred on one theme 'play ball' (i.e. check your testicles) using slang (balls).

- 'Play ball: Testicular cancer is not something that happens to older people.'
- 'Play ball: 'Early diagnosis of testicular cancer is associated with a positive outcome'.
- Q: 'Which is the odd one out? Chlamydia, HIV or testicular cancer? A: Testicular cancer – it's not sexually transmitted.' Play ball.
- 'Everyone play ball: Testicular cancer affects everyone.'

CHAPTER 5

Activity 5.1: Different channels of communication

1   Channels include interpersonal, intrapersonal, organizational and community.
2   Yes.

Activity 5.2: Identifying sub-groups

1   Enjoyment, like, convenience, friends and family eat these foods, easy to cook, cheap.
2   No. See Activity 4.1.

Activity 5.3: Including interpersonal elements

1   Text messaging services, a telephone helpline, email, social networking sites, use peer supporters in local settings.
2   Electronic elements may be set up at a reasonably low cost, essentially the more interaction the more time and resources may be required.

Activity 5.4: Working with myths

1   Incorporate the target group into all campaign messages. Focus on addressing on the main myths in messages and correcting these, such as promoting the ways TB can be transmitted.
2   Messages could be linked to myths. For example, TB is not transmitted through sexual contact.
3   In collaboration with the target group, find media sources that are able to explain things in more detail. Using edutainment or stories for use on the radio is a possibility to encourage interpersonal discussion that promotes correct transmission and facts around TB.

Activity 5.5: Effective uses of media

1   Any news items in the recent news.
2   Any example of media advocacy such as 'The Truth' campaign.
3   Examples include the BHF (2008) 2 minutes campaign available at www.2minutes.org.uk/
4   Examples include Time to change campaign available at www.time-to-change.org.uk/home/

Activity 5.6: Using magazines to promote health

1   One example: In the UK magazines for black women include *Pride, Snoop, Black Hair, Woman to Woman*.
2   Using media advocacy to challenge negative roles models, promoting positive healthy role models using real life stories, images and articles.

Activity 5.7: Advantages and disadvantages of using different media

•   Newspapers are read for longer periods of time, may have higher literacy levels and can have both longer messages and content.
•   Billboards have high visibility and are good for short messages. They can only be accessed by those passing the location and detailed content is not possible.
•   Leaflets are easily distributed but may be easily overlooked or ignored depending on distribution methods. They are usually low cost.
•   Radio reaches specific audiences and not mass groups and is able to use advertisements or content linked into shows i.e. stories or dramas.

Activity 5.8: Adapting information technology for campaigns

1 Customizability could include using email, text-messaging or MSN messenger.
Interconnectivity could be the use of a discussion board.
Confidentiality could be mechanisms that allow users to create a pseudonym.

Activity 5.9: Experimental marketing

1 An example could be: secondary school children from one school and oral hygiene. One experimental setting could be fast food restaurants.
2 Strategies could include 5-minute cooking classes in the car park, free tasters, give-aways such as children's plastic plates with the campaign logo, badges or stickers and re-usable carrier bags.

CHAPTER 6

Activity 6.1: Matching aims to messages

One example:

1 To reduce speed and drive at 20 mph.
2 Why reduce speed, why a school zone and to drive at 20 mph.
3 Instruction message.

Activity 6.2: Gain frame and loss frame messages

1 Gain: You can prevent diabetes by changing your lifestyle and eating foods that have lower levels of sugar.
Loss: You need to reduce sugar and increase your physical activity levels to lower your risk of diabetes.

Activity 6.3 Cultural relevance of materials

1 One example in the UK might be asylum seekers from Central Africa.
2 Possible considerations could be colours, images, tailoring messages to cultural beliefs, religious beliefs or resources that people can access.

Activity 6.4: Concept, category and value judgement words

1 Words like 'plenty', 'liberal' and 'a while' are problem words.
2 Examples:
'Drink at least two litres of water each day to keep your body hydrated.'
'Apply sunscreen at least every two hours when you are in the sun.'
'Wait at least one hour before swimming after you have eaten.'

Activity 6.5: Writing in the active voice and framing messages

1   Example:

- 'You should try and drink a small cup of water at least every hour in the days following your operation.'
- 'If you spend more than an hour at your computer, try and take a break to reduce risks of postural problems.'

Activity: 6.6 SMOG grading of a health resource

1   This will depend on the resource that you have chosen.

Activity 6.7: Turning content into interactive content

1   Examples include: What are the hazards in your job? Have you had your manual handling training within the last year? When are accidents more likely to happen?
2   Accidents are more likely to happen if you are taking medication. True or False? You should have your manual handling training every year. True or False?
3   Examples include a space to write a note of the date when you were last trained. Write down when your training is next due. Write down three reasons why training is important.

Activity 6.8: Designing a leaflet using best practice

One example:

1   Target group (South Asian 1st generation young families) would be involved in all pre-planning.
2   The main aim is: To increase awareness of the hazards in the home associated with childhood accidents under five. This leaflet will concentrate specifically on the kitchen. The main message is to keep children safe in the kitchen by moving household substances i.e. bleach, and sharp objects out of reach, as well as ensuring safe cooking practices.
3   Low grade reading levels will be used. Messages will be framed, e.g. 'It is a good idea if you move cleaning products out of children's reach', and thus use positive framing and active voice.
4   Font size 14, with dark blue on white will be used.
5   Design will use simple question and answer structure and incorporate colours selected by the target group.
6   A space will be left for 'What I will do in my home to keep my children safe ...' as well as a short five question quiz based on the leaflet content.
7   Simple drawing will be used with a cross or tick to indicate good and bad practices.
8   Pre-testing with target group will be undertaken.

CHAPTER 7

Activity 7.1: Identifying challenges to evaluation

1   Locating students, local council advertising and the impacts of cycle lanes.
2   Locate students in classes or common locations, i.e. student union, library and use campus mail shots, advertising or email with incentives.

Specifically link evaluation questions to the university campus campaign, i.e. recall of university messages. Ask in addition if students have seen other messages, i.e. local council ones. Ask why people have started to commute to distinguish between local council and university campaigns.

Activity 7.2: Establishing a baseline or control group

1   The same age group booking with a different travel company in the same location, or the same travel company and same age group in a different country or resort.
2   Pre-testing when holidays are booked or before embarking on holiday, i.e. at the airport.

Activity 7.3: Using formative evaluation

1   Questions include: What they want stickers to look like, when helmets are least likely to be used, barriers and benefits to helmet use as noted by target group.
2   Examples include: In class activities or brief focus groups at lunchtimes or after school. Encourage drawings and paintings to suggest when children should wear helmets.

Activity 7.4: Using process evaluation

1   Questions include: What posters/flyers have you seen and where did you see these? What were the main messages from these? Have you heard of any of the walks? Have you been on any walks? Do you know anyone else that has been on a walk? What might stop you going on a walk? Can you remember the campaign messages?
2   Examples include: Questionnaires or short interviews in local locations, i.e. in the leisure centre, in popular places, i.e. local shopping centre.

Activity 7.5: Using impact evaluation

1   Questions include: Did you receive the email? Can you recall the main message? Did you visit the website? Have you looked for more information on prostate cancer? Do you know the signs of prostate cancer? Did you find the information you needed on the website? Have you been to a medical professional as a result of this information?
2   Examples include: Email brief questionnaire, office door knocking, interviews in staff room, and short postcard style questionnaires with competition incentive.

Activity 7.6: Using outcome evaluation

1   Questions include: Do you feel confident at bathing a new baby? Did the training assist you in bathing a new baby? Did you breastfeed your baby? Have you put any measures into your house for safety? Were these the result of your training? Do you feel the training helped you to cope with being a new parent?
2   Examples include: Postal or telephone questionnaires, interviews face to face, follow-up visits with interviews.

Activity 7.7: Dissemination of findings

1   Health professionals, construction workers, manufacturers, sexual health charities/organizations, government, other factory operators, local government/councils, local residents, condom manufacturers, healthcare practitioners inside and outside South Africa, etc.

2 Paper and internet document. Local findings could be condensed into local media such as newspapers or newsletters.
3 Local newspapers, local reports, internet sites.

Activity 7.8: Evaluation techniques

1 *Process:* Did you attend the exercise session? Do you have the exercises to do at home? Are you doing the exercises at home? Are there any exercises you do not understand? Are you increasing your daily physical activity levels? What are you doing to increase these levels?
Impact: How many times a week have you been doing the exercises? How much more daily physical activity are you doing? Have you fallen during this time? Can you recall the main campaign messages?
Outcome: Are you sustaining the daily exercises? Are you still doing daily physical activity? Have you fallen within the last 6 months? Can you recall the campaign messages?
2 Interviews, face-to-face visits, questionnaires, demonstration of the daily activities, field observations of physical activity.
3 In homes, in local areas where people are physically active, in the clinic.

Activity 7.9: Monitoring a health issue in the news

One example:

1 Alcohol in the media.
Example search terms: Alcohol, drinking, booze, media, newspaper, television.
2–4 Article about media industry and alcohol ban available at www.guardian.co.uk/media/2009/sep/08/ad-ban-devastate-media-industries

  (a) Newspaper article. *The Guardian* newspaper.
  (b) How much money is spent on alcohol advertising and how if alcohol advertising was banned as recommended by BMA, that media companies would lose considerable money.
  (c) 51.
  (d) No photographs. Usual presentation in *Guardian* format.
  (e) Not front page, but has attracted a number of comments from readers.

5 Examples include: Is there any bias? Or whose views are represented? Whose views might be missed?

Activity 7.10: Evaluating a website

1–2 Interactive quiz, make your own porn star movie that promotes condoms and share this with a friend, telephone helpline, email contacts, competitions and social networking site tags.
3 How many people complete the quiz and what age/sex are they? How many people make a film and share it with their friends? Number of emails or telephone calls. Type of emails and telephone calls. Number of people visiting the site. Number of people entering competitions.

Activity 7.11: Unconventional evaluation

Examples:

1 Process: Count the number of people who have heard about the website from a friend or different sources. Encourage target group involvement in the development of the site: ask what

they would do through a competition to make the site better and incorporate the ideas. Have an amnesty of knives/guns and count those handed in.

2   Impact/outcomes: Make a video, write a song or create art work that has the main messages of the campaign.

Glossary

Acculturation   Adapting or adopting a different culture.

Attitude   An evaluation that a person makes about an attitude 'object'. The attitude 'object' could be themselves, other people, issues (i.e. in the media), or objects (i.e. alcohol).

Bebo   A social networking site on the internet.

Belief   The information that a person has about an object or action forms their beliefs.

Blog   An internet page or pages that an individual or organization updates. It often takes a diary format with pictures or entries at frequent points through a time-span.

Bottom-up approach   This assumes that communities or groups know what they want and are involved in all stages of planning and decision making around interventions.

Campaign   A planned, designed and co-ordinated effort to promote a particular cause.

Chat rooms   An internet-based portal where anyone can 'chat' to each other via a mechanism similar to email.

Communication   The act of communicating a message which requires the exchange of information, thoughts or feelings between individuals or groups.

Community-based participatory research (CBPR)   A research process where the community is a partner in the research process, rather than subject of research.

Electronic media   Media such as the internet, mobile phones or computer packages that have an electronic source.

Empowerment   A term usually used to describe a way of working that enables people to develop knowledge or skills to increase control and power over life circumstances.

Enabling factors   Aspects linked to the individual that are objective i.e. skills, wider environment. Part of the PRECEDE-PROCEED model.

Evaluation   The process by which worth or value of something is decided involving measurement, observation and comparison with the programme/policy aim.

Evidence-based practice   The use of research evidence to guide practice.

Experimental marketing   The use of marketing activities to complement a campaign that have not necessarily been proved effective but are designed to appeal to the audience on a small scale, i.e. setting up physical activity zones for children in a shopping centre.

Extended Parallel Process Model   A theoretical model that includes the variables of attitude, behaviour, intention and efficacy that is linked to the fear appeal approach.

Facebook   A social networking site on the internet.

Fear appeal   A message that contains a threat or other element designed to increase fear of an issue.

Formative evaluation   The pre-evaluation of the main materials and strategies of a campaign before the campaign commences.

Health Belief Model   A model of behavioural change that focuses on an individual weighing up the risks and benefits of behaviours.

Health education   Providing information through constructed opportunities that improve knowledge or skills and increase healthy behaviours.

Health literacy   The ability to locate and understand and act upon basic health information.

Health promotion   The process of enabling people to increase control over their health.

Holistic   A term that includes the wider definition of health including physical mental, social and spiritual health.

HPV   Human papillomavirus (HPV) which is linked to cervical cancer in women.

Impact evaluation   The immediate effects of the campaign.

Intrapersonal communication   Communication at an individual level such as one-to-one.

Inequalities (in health)   Differences in health status between populations or sections of the population.

Information technology   Generally includes all interactive media, i.e. CD ROMs, the internet, touch screen kiosks or computers.

Interpersonal communication   Communication at person-to-person level such as communication between friends, family and peers.

Intervention Mapping (IM)   A famework that can be used for planning an intervention or campaign.

Malaria   A fever caused by a protozoan parasite transmitted through a mosquito bite.

Mass media   Any type of printed or electronic communication medium that is sent to the population at large. It has four main categories: audio-visual broadcast media, audio-visual non-broadcast media, print media and electronic media.

Message framing   The presentation of a message in terms of gains or losses associated with that behaviour.

Model   A simplified version of a theoretical construct.

Monolithic   A single thing that is uniform.

MRSA Methicillin-resistant Staphylococcus aureus infection that is generally present in hospitals or the community. Its spread can be reduced by thorough hand-washing practices.

Narrative The use of stories in such as fictional or factual stories.

Need What a person wants or expresses. There are generally four types of need: normative, comparative, felt and expressed as identified by Bradshaw (1972).

New media New technology that is currently still evolving such as internet-based social networking sites, blogs, SMS on mobile phones.

News item A story, article or piece of news in a paper, magazine or via audio-visual media such as radio or television.

Outpatient A person who accesses services independently and is not resident at a hospital or other medical establishment.

Outcome evaluation The more long-term effects of the campaign. Feedback is the distribution of the campaign's findings back into the evidence base.

Perceived behavioural control The perception a person has of their ability to control an element of their behaviour.

PRECEDE-PROCEED PROCEED stands for Policy, Regulatory and Organizational Constructs in Educational and Environmental Development. PRECEDE stands for Predisposing, Reinforcing and Enabling Constructs in Educational/Ecological Diagnosis and Evaluation.

Predisposing factors Individual characteristics (i.e. attitudes, beliefs). Part of the PRECEDE-PROCEED model.

Process evaluation An evaluation of the implementation of the campaign process which looks to measure the program progress.

Program A planned activity that results in an outcome, similar in format to a campaign.

Public health A societal effort to prevent disease and prolong life.

Public service announcement (PSA) Usually government- or organization-funded messages that are read, printed or screened for free or at a discounted rate on different media channels.

Readability The levels of accessibility of text (i.e. reading grade level of materials).

Reinforcing factors The perceived benefits, barriers, rewards, or punishments as a consequence of performing a behaviour. Part of the PRECEDE-PROCEED model.

Role-play An education method where a person 'acts' a response to a situation. The audience will then 'model' this same response in a real-life situation.

SAM Suitability and assessment of materials (SAM) formula that can be applied to health-related resources.

Screening The procedure for the identification of a certain disease (i.e. breast cancer) to enable early detection and treatment of the disease.

Settings A location where people conduct their lives in work, rest or play that can be a possible influence on health or a location to promote health such as a school or workplace.

Social support   The support received by someone from friends, family or peers.

Social cognitive theory   A behaviour change theory used in health-related disciplines.

Social marketing   A combination of marketing strategies that can be applied to a range of health issues.

Social networking sites   Internet sites created for the purposes of a common interest such as a health issue (a cancer group), or a leisure interest (music) or a friendship network. These can be individually held or run by a group. These currently include sites such as Facebook, Twitter and Bebo.

SMOG   A simple measure of gobbledygook (SMOG) that can be applied to health education materials to identify their readability levels.

SMS messaging   The facility of sending short messages via a mobile phone more commonly called text messaging.

STI   Sexually Transmitted Infection such as HIV, chlamydia or gonorrhoea.

Strategy   A plan of campaign elements such as methods and the delivery of these that will be used in the final campaign.

Stroke   A disabling attack or loss of consciousness due to an interruption of blood flowing to the brain.

Subjective norm   What influential people such as friends and family think and say about a variable (e.g. tobacco smoking) that influences a person.

Tailoring   Adapting information for a specific group of people to fit their individual needs and preferences.

Targeting   Adapting information for a specific group of people based upon group characteristics (see tailoring).

Theory   A set of ideas or arguments that help to understand behaviour in a more simplified way.

Theory of Planned Behaviour   A theoretical model based on the stages a person goes through when changing a behaviour including perceived behavioural control.

Top-down approach   An approach which is dictated by those with power that does not directly include the target group or receivers of the intervention (see Bottom-up approach).

Transtheoretical Model or 'stages of change' model   A stage-step model based on the stages people go through when making a change in their behaviour.

Tweens   A term sometimes applied to an age group of 9-13-year-olds who are not yet 'teenagers', and not really children. They are 'in between'.

Twitter   A social networking site on the internet.

Typography   The style of type used in a resource, i.e. font size, italics, bold.

YouTube   An internet-based site where videos, television advertisements or other visual clips can be viewed.

Values   Acquired by the social world they can influence attitudes and behaviour.

References

Aarø, L E, Flisher, A J, Kaaya, S, Onya, H, Fuglesang, M, Kleep, K et al. (2006) Promoting sexual and reproductive health in early adolescence in South Africa and Tanzania: development of a theory- and evidence-based intervention programme. *Scandinavian Journal of Public Health* 34 (2) 150–158.

Abercrombie, L, Sallis, J, Conway, T, Frank, L, Saelens, B & Chapman, J (2008) Income and racial disparities in access to public parks and private recreation facilities. *American Journal of Preventive Medicine* 34 (1) 9–15.

Abraham, C, Southby, L, Quandte, S, Krahe, B & van der Sluijs, W (2007) What's in a leaflet? Identifying research-based persuasive messages in European alcohol-education leaflets. *Psychology and Health* 22 (1) 31–60.

Abroms, L C & Lefebure, R C (2009) Obama's wired campaign: lessons for public health communication. *Journal of Health Communication* 14 (5) 415–423.

Ackard, D M & Neumark-Sztainer, C (2001) Health care information sources for adolescents: age and gender difference on use, concerns and needs. *Journal of Adolescent Health* 29 (3) 170–176.

Adams, J, Witten, K & Conway, K (2009) Community development as health promotion: evaluating a complex locality-based project in New Zealand. *Community Development Journal* 44 (2) 140–157.

Ajzen, I (1980) *Understanding attitudes and predicting social behaviour*. Prentice-Hall, Upper Saddle River, NJ.

Ajzen, I (1991) The Theory of Planned Behaviour. *Organisational Behaviour and Human Decision Processes* 50 179–211, available at www-unix.oit.umass.edu/~aizen/index.html

Alcorn, K (2005) *Stigma and myths still harming TB fight. Aids Map News*. Tue 25 Oct., available at www.aidsmap.com/en/news/F1064B98-5293-4636-85F0-14D07AA15DD2. asp

Andersen, P A, Buller, D B, Walkosz, B J, Maloy, J, Scott, M D, Cutter, D R et al. (2009) Testing a theory based health communication program: a replication of Go Sun Smart in outdoor winter recreation. *Journal of Health Communication* 14 (4) 346–365.

Andreeva, V A, Reynolds, K D, Buller, D B, Chou, C P & Yaroch, A L (2008) Concurrent psychosocial predictors of sun safety among middle school youth. *The Journal of School Health* 78 (7) 374–381.

Annett, H & Rifkin, S B (1995) *Guidelines for rapid participatory appraisals to assess community health needs: a focus on health improvements for low-income urban and rural areas*. World Health Organization, Geneva.

Apollonio, D E & Malone, R E (2009) Turning negative into positive: public health media campaigns and negative advertising. *Health Education Research* 24 (3) 483–495.

Arden, M A & Armitage, C J (2008) Predicting and explaining transtheoretical model stage transitions in relation to condom-carrying behaviour. *British Journal of Health Psychology* 13 (4) 719–735.

Artienza, A A, Yaroch, A L, Masse, L G, Moser, R P, Hesse, B W & King, A C (2006) Identifying sedentary sub-groups. The National Cancer Institute's health information national trends survey. *American Journal of Preventive Medicine* 31 (5) 383–390.

Atkin, C (2001) *Theory and principles of media health campaigns*. 49–68 in Rice, R E & Atkin, C K (eds) *Public communication campaigns, 3rd edition*. Sage, London.

Atkin, C K & Freimuth, V S (2001) *Formative evaluation research in campaign design* 125–145 in Rice, R E & Atkin, C K (eds) *Public communication campaigns, 3rd edition*. Sage, London.

Atun, R A & Sittampalam, S R (2006) A review of the characteristics and benefits of SMS in delivering healthcare. *The Vodafone Policy Paper Series*. 4 (March) 18–28, available at www.vodafone.com

Aubel, J, Toure, I & Diagne, M (2004) Senegalese grandmothers promote improved nutrition practice: the guardians of tradition are not adverse to change. *Social Science and Medicine* 59 (5) 945–959.

Aveyard, P, Massey, L, Parsons, A, Manaseki, S & Griffin, C (2009) The effect of the Transtheoretical model based interventions on smoking cessation. *Social Science and Medicine* 68 (3) 397–403.

Baker, A (2009) Alcohol related deaths by occupation: what do data for England and Wales in 2001–2005 tell us about doctors' mortality? *Alcohol and Alcholism* 43 (2) 121–122.

Bandura, A (1988) Organizational application of Social Cognitive Theory. *Australian Journal of Management* 13 (2) 275–302.

Barker, K L, Minns Lowe, C J & Reid, M (2007) The development and use of mass media interventions for health-care messages about back pain: what do members of the public think? *Manual Therapy* 12 (4) 335–341.

Bartholomew, L K, Parcel, G S, Kok, G & Gottlieb, N H (2001) Intervention mapping. In *Designing theory and evidence based health promotion programs*. McGraw-Hill, New York.

Bartholomew, L K, Parcel, G S, Kok, G & Gottlieb, N H (2006) *Planning health promotion programs an intervention mapping approach*. Jossey-Bass, San Francisco, CA.

Bastian, H (2008) Health literacy and patient information: developing the methodology for a national evidence-based health website. *Patient Education and Counseling* 73 (3) 551–556.

Bauman, A, Smith, B J, Maibach, E W & Reger-Nash, P (2006) Evaluation of mass media information for physical activity. *Evaluation and Program Planning* 29 (3) 312–322.

Beck, K (2009) Lessons learned from evaluating Maryland's drunk driving campaign: assessing the evidence for cognitive and behavioural and public health impact. *Health Promotion Practice* 10 (3) 370–377.

Becker, M H (1974) The Health Belief Model and personal health behaviour. *Health Education Monographs* 2 (4) 324–473.

Berry, T R, Spence, J C, Plotnikoff, R C, Bauman, A, McCargar, L, Witcher, C et al. (2009) A mixed methods evaluation of televised health promotion advertisements targeted at older adults. *Evaluation and Program Planning* 32 (3) 278–288.

Bessinger, R, Katende, C & Gupta, N (2004) Multimedia campaign exposure effects on knowledge and use of condoms for STI and HIV/AIDS prevention in Uganda. *Evaluation and Program Planning* 27 (4) 397–407.

Best, A, Stokols, D, Green, L W, Leischow, S, Holmes, B & Buchholz, K (2003) An integrative framework for community partnering to translate theory into effective health promotion strategy. *American Journal of Health Promotion* 18 (2) 168–176.

Boer, H & Mashamba, M T (2007) Gender power imbalance and different psychosocial correlates of intended condom use among male and female adolescents from Venda, South Africa. *British Journal of Health Psychology* 21 (1) 51–63.

Boniface, D R, Cottee, M J, Neal, D & Skinner, A (2001) Social and demographic factors predictive of change over seven years in CHD related behaviours in men aged 18–49 years. *Public Health* 115 (4) 246–252.

Bos, A E R, Schaalma, H P & Pryor, J B (2008) Reducing AIDS-related stigma in developing countries: the importance of theory and evidence based interventions. *Psychology, Health and Medicine* 13 (4) 450–460.

Bosmans, M, Cikuru, M N, Claeys, P & Temmerman, M (2006) Where have all the condoms gone in adolescent programmes in the Democratic Republic of Congo? *Reproductive Health Matters* 14 (28) 80–88.

Bradshaw, J (1972) A taxonomy of social need. *New Society* (March) 640–643.

British Heart Foundation (BHF) (2009) *yoobots* available at www.yoobot.co.uk/

British Heart Foundation (BHF) (2008) *2 Minutes* available at www.2minutes.org.uk/

Brown, C S, Lloyd, S & Murray, S A (2006) Using consecutive rapid participatory appraisal studies to assess, facilitate and evaluate health and social change in community settings. *BMC Public Health*, Mar 15 6 (68), available at www.biomedcentral.com/1471-2458/6/68

Brug, J, Oenema, A & Ferreira, I (2005) Theory, evidence and intervention mapping to improve behaviour nutrition and physical activity interventions. *International Journal of Behavioural Nutrition and Physical Activity* 2 (2), available at http://www.ijbnpa.org/content/2/1/2

Brunton, G, Rees, R & Bonnell, C (2007) *Reviewing the evidence base for health promotion planning*, 37–58, in Macdowall, W, Bonell, C & Davies, M *Health promotion practice*, Open University Press, Maidenhead.

Bryne, M & Curtis, R (2000) Designing health communication: testing the explanations for the impact of communication medium on effectiveness. *British Journal of Health Psychology* 5 (2) 189–199.

Buckley, C, Barrett, J & Adkins, K (2008) Reproductive health information for young women in Kazakhstan: disparities in access by channel. *Journal of Health Communication* 13 (7) 681–697.

Bull, F C, Holt, C L, Kreuter, M W, Clark, E M & Scharff, D (2001) Understanding the effects of printed health education materials: which features lead to which outcomes? *Journal of Health Communication* 6 (3) 265–279.

Bust, P D, Gibb, A G F & Pink, S (2008) Managing construction health and safety: migrant workers and communicating safety messages. *Safety Science* 46 (4) 585–602.

Byrd, T L, Peterson, S K, Chavez, R & Heckert, A (2004) Cervical screening beliefs among young Hispanic women. *Preventive Medicine* 38 (2) 192–197.

Calabro, K, Taylor, W C & Kapadia, A (1996) Pregnancy, alcohol use and the effectiveness of written health education materials. *Patient Education and Counseling* 29 (3) 301–309.

Cameron, E, Mathers, J & Parry, J (2008) 'Health and well-being': questioning the use of health concepts in public health policy and practice. *Critical Public Health* 18 (2) 225–232.

Campo, S, Askelson, N M, Routsong, T, Graaf, L J, Losch, M & Smoth, H (2008) The Green Acres Effect: the need for a new colorectal cancer screening campaign tailored to rural audiences. *Health Education and Behaviour* 35 (6) 749–762.

Cancer Research UK (2009) *CancerChat*, available at www.cancerchat.org.uk

Caperchione, C M, Duncan, M J, Mummery, K, Steele, R & Schofield, G (2008) Mediating relationship between body mass index and the direct measures of the theory of Planned Behaviour on physical activity intention. *Psychology, Health and Medicine* 13 (2) 168–179.

CBS Outdoor (2009a) *Inspire me gallery* www.cbsoutdoor.co.uk/Inspire-me/Gallery/

CBS Outdoor (2009b) *Audience*, available at www.cbsoutdoor.co.uk

CBS Outdoor (2009c) *Ten reasons to use bus advertising*, available at www.cbsoutdoor.co.uk

Centre for Communicable Diseases (CDC) (2009) *VERB youth campaign,* available at www.cdc.gov/youthcampaign/index.htm

Centers for Disease Control and Prevention (CDC) (1999) *Scientific and technical information: simply put 2nd edition.* CDC, Atlanta, Georgia.

Champion, V L, Monahan, P O, Springston, J K, Russell, K, Zollinter, T W, Saywell, R M et al. (2008) Measuring mammography and breast cancer beliefs in African American women. *Journal of Health Psychology* 13 (6) 827–837.

Chang, C (2009) Psychological motives versus health concerns: predicting smoking attitudes and promoting antismoking attitudes. *Health Communication* 24 (11) 1–11.

Chinn, D J, White, M, Howel, D, Harland, J O E & Drinkwater, C K (2006) Factors associated with non-participation in a physical activity promotion trial. *Public Health* 120 (4) 309–319.

Clements, A, Parry-Langdon, N & Roberts, C (2006) Men's health – is there a popular press potential? *Health Education Journal* 65 (3) 277–287.

Coffman, J (2002) *Public communication campaign evaluation: an environmental scan of challenges, criticisms, practice and opportunities.* Harvard Family Research Project, Cambridge, MA.

Coleman, L & Testa, A (2007) Sexual health knowledge, attitudes and behaviours among an ethnically diverse sample of young people in the UK. *Health Education Journal* 66 (3) 68–81.

Community Restorative Centre (NSW) *Jailbreak radio,* available at www.crcnsw.org.au/services/Jailbreak.htm

Condoms essential wear (2009) *Condoms essential wear,* available at www.condomessentialwear.co.uk

Corcoran, N (2007a) Mass media in health communication 73–95 in Corcoran, N (ed.) *Communicating health: strategies for health promotion.* Sage, London.

Corcoran, S (2007b) Evidence based practice and communication 139–159, in Corcoran, N (ed.) *Communicating health: strategies for health promotion.* Sage, London.

Corcoran, N (2007c) Theories and models in communicating health messages, 5–31, in Corcoran, N (ed.) *Communicating health: strategies for health promotion.* Sage, London.

Corcoran, N (2008) How can social marketing be used to promote sport? *London Journal of Sport, Tourism and Creative Industries* 1 (1), available at http://blogs.londonmet.ac.uk/ljtsci/2008/11/16/corcoran-how-can-social-marketing-be-used-to-promote-sport/

Corcoran, N & Bone, A (2007) Using settings to communicate health promotion, 117–138, in Corcoran, N (ed.) *Communicating health: strategies for health promotion.* Sage, London.

Corcoran, N & Corcoran S (2007) Social and psychological factors in communication, 32–52, in Corcoran, N (ed.) *Communicating health strategies for health promotion.* Sage, London.

Corcoran, N & Garlick, J (2007) Evidence based practice and communication, 139–158, in Corcoran, N (ed.) *Communicating health: strategies for health promotion.* Sage, London.

Cotton, S & Gupta, S (2004) Characteristics of online and offline health information seeks and factors that discriminate between them. *Social Science and Medicine* 59 (9) 1795–1806.

Courtenay, W H, Mccreary, D R & Merighi, J R (2002) Gender and ethnic differences in health beliefs and behaviour. *Journal of Health Psychology* 7 (3) 219–231.

Cristancho, S, Garces, D M, Peters, K E, Mueller, B C (2008) Listening to Rural Hispanic immigrants in the Midwest: a community-based participatory assessment of major barriers to health care access and use. *Qualitative Health Research* 18 (5) 633–646.

Cropley, L (2004) The effect of health education interventions on child malaria treatment-seeking practices among mothers in rural refugee villages in Belize, Central America. *Health Promotion International* 19 (4) 445–452.

Cunningham, W E, Davidson, P L, Nakazone, T T & Andersen, R M (1999) Do black and white adults use the same sources of information about AIDS prevention? *Health Education and Behaviour* 26 (5) 703–713.

D'Silva, M U & Palmgreen, P (2007) Individual differences and context: factors mediating recall of anti-drug public service announcements. *Health Communication* 21 (1) 65–71.

Davies, M & Macdowall, W (eds) (2006) *Health promotion theory.* Open University Press, Maidenhead.

Dearing, J W, Maibach, E W & Butler, D B (2006) A convergent diffusion and social marketing approach for disseminating proven approaches to physical activity promotion. *American Journal of Preventive Medicine* 31 (4s) s11–s23.

Delre, S A, Jager, W, Bijmout, T H A & Janssen, M A (2007) Targeting and timing promotional activities: an agent-based model for the take off of new products. *Journal of Business Research* 60 (8) 826–835.

Delvin, K (2008) Jamie Oliver approach beats public health campaigns claims psychologist, 26 Nov 08, 7.33 GMT, available at www.telegraph.co.uk/health/healthnews

De Nooijer, J, Lechner, L & de Vries, H (2002) Tailored versus general information on early detection of cancer: a comparison of the reactions of Dutch adults and the impact on attitudes and behaviours. *Health Education Research* 17 (2) 239–252.

De Vet, E, De Nooijer, J, De Vries, N K & Brug, J (2008) Do the transtheoretical processes of change predict transitions in stages of change for fruit intake? *Health Education and Behaviour* 35 (5) 603–618.

Department of Health (2009) *Change4Life*, available at www.nhs.uk/change4life

Department of Health (2004) *Choosing health: making healthy choices easier.* The Stationery Office, London, available at www.dh.gov.uk

Department for Transport (DfT) (2009a) *Think*, available at www.dft.gov.uk/think

Department for Transport (DfT) (2009b) *Drug driving: the facts*, available at www.dft.gov.uk/think/focusareas/driving/drugdriving

Department of Transport (DfT) (2009c) *Campaign calendar*, available at http://think.dft.gov.uk/think/mediacentre/calendar

Department for Transport (DfT) (2009d) *Live with it*, available at www.dft.gov.uk/think

Department for Transport (DfT) (2009e) *Tales of the road*, available at www.talesoftheroad.direct.gov.uk

Diabetes UK (2009) *Our 2 minute test*, available at www.diabetes.org.uk/measure%2Dup/

Doak, C C, Doak, L C & Root, J H (1996) *Teaching patients with low literacy skills, 2nd edition*. Lippincott Company, Philadelphia, available at www.hsph.harvard.edu/health-literacy/doak.html

Dobbinson, S J, Wakefield, M A, Jansen, K M, Herd, N L, Spittal, M J, Lipscomb, J E et al. (2008) Weekend sun protection and sunburn in Australia. Trends 1987–2002 and association with SunSmart advertising. *American Journal of Preventive Medicine* 34 (2) 94–101.

Dodds, C (2002) Messages of responsibility: HIV/AIDS prevention materials in England. *Health* 6 (2) 139–171.

Douglas, J, Lloyd, C, & Sidell, M (2007) Using research to plan multi-disciplinary public health interventions, 297–326 in Earle, S, Lloyd, C, Sidell, M & Spurr, S (eds) *Theory and research in promoting public health*. Sage/The Open University, London.

Duan, N, Fox, S, Pitkin, K, Derose, K, Carson, S & Stockdale, S (2005) Identifying churches for community-based mammography promotion: lessons from the LAMP study. *Health Education and Behaviour* 32 (4) 536–548.

Duerksen, S C, Mikail, A, Tom, L, Patton, A, Lopez, J, Amador, X et al (2005) Health disparities and advertising content of women's magazines: a cross-sectional study. *BMC Public Health*, 5:85, available at www.biomedcentral.com/1471-458/5/85

DuRant, R H, Wolfson, M, LaFrance, B, Balkrishnan, R & Altman, D (2006) An evaluation of mass media campaign to encourage parents of adolescents to talk to their children about sex. *Journal of Adolescent Health* 38 298.e1–298.e9.

Dutta-Bergman, M J (2005) Theory and practice in health communication campaigns: a critical interrogation. *Health Communication* 18 (2) 103–122.

Dutton, G R, Provost, B C, Tan, F & Smith, D (2008) A tailored print-based physical activity intervention for patients with type 2 diabetes. *Preventive Medicine* 47 (4) 409–411.

Duyn, M A S, McCrae, T, Wingrove, B K, Henderson, K M, Boyd, J K, Kawaga-Singer, M, et al. (2007) Adapting evidence based strategies to increase physical activity among African-Americans, Hispanics, Hmong and Native Hawaiians: a social marketing approach: preventing chronic disease. *Public Health Research, Practice and Policy* 4 (4) 1–11.

Dyer, K J, Fearon, K L H, Buckner, K & Richardson, R A (2005) Diet and colorectal cancer risk: evaluation of a nutritional leaflet. *Health Education Journal* 64 (3) 247–255.

Elliott, J (2009) The Jade Goody effect on screening, BBC News, Wed 22 Mar, available at http://news.bbc.co.uk/1/hi/health/7925685.stm

Evans, W D, Blitstein, J, Hessey, J C, Renaud, J & Yaroch, A L (2008) Systematic review of public health branding. *Journal of Health Communication* 13 (8) 721–741.

Evans, W D, Uhrig, J, Davis, K & McCormack, L (2009) Efficacy methods to evaluate health communication and marketing campaigns. *Journal of Health Communication* 14 (4) 315–330.

Evans, W D, Wasserman, J, Bertolotti, E & Martine, S (2002) Branding behaviour: the strategy behind the truth campaign. *Social Marketing Quarterly* VIII (3) 17–29.

Evers, K E, Prochaska, J O, Driskell, M, Cummins, C O & Velicer, W F (2003) Strengths and weaknesses of health behaviour change programs on the internet. *Journal of Health Psychology* 8 (1) 63–70.

Evers, K E, Prochaska, J O, Van Marter, D F, Johnson, J L & Prochaska, J M (2007) Transtheoretical based bullying prevention effectiveness trials in middle schools and high schools. *Educational Research* 49 (4) 397–414.

Eyles, P, Skelly, J & Schmuck, M (2003) Evaluating patient choice of typeface style and font size for written health information in an outpatient setting. *Clinical Effectiveness in Nursing* 7 (2) 94–98.

Facefront (2009) *Theatre in education*, available at www.facefront.org

Farquhar, S A, Parker, E A, Schulz, A J & Israel, B A (2006) Application of qualitative methods in program planning for health promotion interventions. *Health Promotion Practice* 7 (2) 234–242.

Farr, A C, Witte, K & Jarato, K (2005) The effectiveness of media use in health education: evaluation of a HIV/AIDS radio campaign in Ethiopia. *Journal of Health Communication* 10 (3) 225–235.

Federici, A, Barca, A, Baiocchi, D, Quadrino, F, Valle, S, Borgia, P et al. (2008) Can colorectal cancer mass-screening organization be evidence-based? Lessons from failures: the experimental and pilot phases of the Lazio program. *BMC Public Health* (8) 318–328, available at www.biomedcentral.com/1471-2458/8/318

Ferrand, C, Perrin, C & Nassare, S (2008) Motives for regular physical activity in women and men: a qualitative study in French adults with type 2 diabetes belonging to a patients association. *Health and Social Care in the Community* 16 (5) 511–520.

Fishbein, M & Cappella, J N (2006) The role of theory in developing effective communications. *Journal of Communication* 56 (s1) s1–s17.

Fishbein, M & Yzer, M C (2003) Using theory to develop effective health behaviour interventions. *Communication Theory* 13 (2) 164–183.

Fjeldsoe, B S, Marshall, A L & Miller, Y D (2009) Behaviour change interventions delivered by mobile telephoning short message service. *American Journal of Preventive Medicine* 36 (2) 165–173.

Flisher, A J, Myer, L, Mèrais, A, Lombard, C & Reddy, P (2007) Prevalence and correlates of partner violence among South African adolescents. *Journal of Child Psychology and Psychiatry* 48 (6) 619–627.

Flynn, B S, Worden, J K, Bunn, T Y, Dorwaldt, A L, Connolly, S W & Ashikaa, T (2007) Youth audience segmentation strategies for smoking prevention mass media campaigns based on message appeal. *Health Education Behaviour* 34 (4) 578–593.

Friedman, D B, Hoffman-Goetz, L (2006) A systematic review of readability and comprehension instruments used for print and web-based cancer information. *Health Education and Behaviour* 33 (3) 352–373.

Friedman, D B & Hoffman-Goetz, L (2007) An exploratory study of older adults' comprehension of printed cancer information: is readability a key factor? *Journal of Health Communication* 12 (5) 423–437.

Gallivan, J, Lising, M, Ammary, N J & Gremberg, R (2007) The national diabetes education programs' 'Control your diabetes for life' campaign: design, implementation and lessons learned. *Social Marketing Quarterly* XIII (4) 65–82.

Gao, W, DeSouza, R, Paterson, J & Lu, T (2008) Factors affecting uptake of cervical cancer screening among Chinese women in New Zealand. *International Journal of Gynecology and Obstetrics* 103 (1) 76–82.

Gazabon, S A, Morokoff, P J, Harlow, L L, Ward, R M & Quina, K (2007) Applying the transtheoretical model to ethnically diverse women at risk for HIV. *Health Education & Behavior* 34 (2) 297–314.

Gerend, M A & Cullen, M (2008) Effects of message framing and temporal context on college student drinking behaviour. *Journal of Experimental Social Psychology* 44 (4) 1167–1173.

Gerend, M A, Shepherd, J E & Monday, K A (2008) Behavioral frequency moderates the effects of message framing on HPV vaccine acceptability. *Annals of Behavioural Medicine* 35 (2) 221–229.

Godin, G, Gagnon, H, Alary, M, Levy, J L & Otis, J (2007) The degree of planning: an indicator of the potential success of health education programs. *Promotion and Education* 14 (3) 138–172.

Goldman, K D & Schmalz, K J (2007) 'As you likert it': Conducting gap based needs assessments. *Health Promotion Practice* 8 (3) 225–228.

Gordon, R, McDermott, L, Stead, M, Angus, K & Hastings, G (2006) *A review of the effectiveness of social marketing physical activity interventions. NSCM report 1.* National Social Marketing Centre for Excellence, London.

Gould, D and Company (2004) *Writing a media analysis*, available at www.mediaevaluationproject.org/WorkingPaper2.pdf

Gratton, L, Povey, R & Clark-Carter, D (2007) Promoting children's fruit and vegetable consumption: interventions using the theory of planned behaviour as a framework. *British Journal of Health Psychology* 12 (4) 639–650.

Gray, N J, Klein, J D, Noyce, P R, Hesselberg, T S & Cantrill, J A (2005) Health information seeking behaviour in adolescents: the place of the internet. *Social Science and Medicine* 60 (7) 1467–1478.

Green, E C & Witte, K (2006) Can fear arousal in public health campaigns contribute to the decline of HIV prevalence? *Journal of Health Communication* 11 (3) 245–259.

Green, L W (2000) The role of theory in evidence based health promotion practice editorial. *Health Education Research* 15 (2) 125–129.

Green, L W and Kreuter, M W (2005) *Health promotion planning: an educational and ecological approach, 3rd edition*. McGraw-Hill, London.

Gregg, J & O'Hara, L (2007) The red lotus model for health promotion: a new model for holistic, ecological, salutogenic health promotion practice. *Health Promotion Journal of Australia* 18 (1) 12–19.

Gwent Police and Tredegar Comprehensive School (2009) Cow – the film that will stop you texting and driving, available at www.youtube.com/watch?v=KF0_7qC6YFo

Halder, A K, Tiro, J A, Glassman, B, Rakowski, W, Fernandez, M E, Perez, C A et al. (2008) Lessons learned from developing a tailored print intervention: a guide for practitioners and researchers new to tailoring. *Health Promotion Practice* 9 (3) 281–288.

Hall, B, Howard, K & McCafferty, K (2008) Do cervical cancer screening patient information leaflets meet the HPV information needs of women? *Patient Education and Counseling* 72 (1) 78–87.

Harmon, A H, Grim, B J & Gromis, J C (2007) Improving nutrition education newsletters for the food stamp eligible audience. *Health Promotion Practice* 8 (4) 394–402.

Harrison, K & Bond, B J (2007) Gaming magazines and the drive for muscularity in pre-adolescent boys: a longitudinal examination. *Body Image* 4 (3) 269–277.

Heinen, M M, Bartholomew, L K, Wensign, M, Kerkhof, P & Achterberg, T (2006) Supporting adherence and healthy lifestyles in leg ulcer patients: systematic development of the Lively Legs program for dermatology outpatient clinics. *Patient Education and Counselling* 61(2) 279–291.

Heitzler, C D, Ashbury, L C & Kusner, S L (2008) Bringing 'play' to life: the use of experimental marketing in the VERB™ campaign. *American Journal of Preventive Medicine* 34 (6s) s188–193.

Hemmick, R S & McCarthy, S K (2007) Provision of emergency contraceptive pills at college and university students health centres in Florida. *Journal of Adolescent Health* 40 (1) 92–95.

Hill, C & Abraham, C (2008) School-based, randomised controlled trial of an evidence-based condom promotion leaflet. *Psychology and Health* 23 (1) 41–56.

Hill, C, Abraham, C & Wright, D B (2007) Can theory based messages in combination with cognitive prompts promote exercise in classroom settings? *Social Science and Medicine* 65 (5) 1049–1058.

Hinyard, L J & Kreuter, M W (2007) Using narrative communication as a tool for health behaviour change: a conceptual theoretical and empirical overview. *Health Education and Behaviour* 34 (5) 777–792.

Hoa, N P, Chuc, N T K & Thorson, A (2009) Knowledge, attitudes and practices about tuberculosis and choice of communication channels in a rural community in Vietnam. *Health Policy* 90 (1) 8–12.

Hoeken, H, Swanepoel, P, Saal, E & Jansen, C (2009) Using message form to stimulate conversations: the case of Tropes. *Communication Theory* 19 (1) 49–65.

Hoffman, T & McKenna, K (2006) Analysis of stroke patients' and carers' reading ability and the content and design of written materials: recommendations for improving written stroke information. *Patient Education and Counseling* 60 (3) 286–293.

Hoffman, T & Worrall, L (2004) Designing effective written health education materials: considerations for health professionals. *Disability and Rehabilitation* 26 (19) 1166–1173.

Holzner, B M & Oetomo, D (2004) Youth, sexuality and sex education messages in Indonesia: issues of desire and control. *Reproductive Health Matters* 12 (23) 40–49.

Hooker, S P, Cirill, L A & Geraghty, A (2009) Evaluation of the walkable neighborhoods for seniors project in Sacramento County. *Health Promotion Practice* 10 (3) 402–410.

Horst, C, Chasela, C, Ahmed, Y, Hoffman, I, Hosseinipour, M, Knight, R, et al. (2009) Modifications of a large HIV prevention clinical trial to fit changing realities: a case study of the Breastfeeding, Antiretroviral and Nutrition (BAN) protocol in Lilongwe, Malawi. *Contemporary Clinical Trials* 30 (1) 24–33.

Hou, S, Fernandez, M E & Parcel, G S (2004) Development of a cervical cancer educational program for Chinese women using intervention mapping. *Health Promotion Practice* 5 (1) 80–87.

Houts, P S, Doak, C C, Doak, L G & Loscalzo, M J (2006) The role of pictures in improving health communication: a review of research on attention, comprehension, recall and adherence. *Patient Education and Counseling* 61 (1) 173–190.

Hunter, C M, Peterson, A L, Alvarez, L M, Poston, W C, Brundige, A R, Haddock, C K et al. (2008) Weight management using the internet: a randomized control trial. *American Journal of Preventive Medicine* 34 (2) 119–126.

Iriyama, S, Nakahara, S, Jimba, M, Ichikawa, M & Wakai, S (2007) AIDS health beliefs and intention for sexual abstinence among male adolescent students in Kathmandu, Nepal: a test of perceived severity and susceptibility. *Public Health* 121 (1) 64–72.

Jans, M, Proper, K & Hildebrant, V (2007) Sedentary behaviours in Dutch workers: differences between occupations and business sectors. *American Journal of Preventive Medicine* 33 (6) 450–454.

JC Decaux (2009) Campaign gallery, available at www.jcdecaux.co.uk/campaigngallery/

Jilcott, S B, Laraia, B A, Evenson, K R, Lowenstein, L M & Ammerman, A S (2007) A guide for developing intervention tools addressing environmental factors to improve diet and physical activity. *Health Promotion Practice* 8 (2) 192–204.

Johnson, S S, Paiva, A L, Cummins, C O, Johnson, J L, Dyment, S J, Wright et al. (2008) Transtheoretical model-based multiple behaviour intervention for weight management: effectiveness on a population basis. *Preventive Medicine* 46 (3) 238–246.

Kahan, B & Goodstadt, M (2002) *The IDM manual: introduction and basics.* Centre for health promotion, University of Toronto, Toronto.

Kaler, A (2009) Health interventions and the persistence of rumour: the circulation of sterility stories in African public health campaigns. *Social Science and Medicine* 68 (9) 1711–1719.

Karayurt, O, Ozmen, D & Cetinkayai, A (2008) Awareness of breast cancer risk factors and practice of breast self examination among high school students in Turkey. *BMC Public Health*, 08 359, available at www.biomedcentral.com/content/pdf/1471-2458-8-359.pdf

Kari, H K (2006) Availability and accessibility of ITC in the rural communities of Nigeria. *The electronic library* 25 (3) 363–372.

Kerr, J, Eves, F F & Carroll, D (2001) Getting more people on the stairs: the impact of a new message format. *Journal of Health Psychology* 6 (5) 495–500.

Kerr-Corrêa, F, Igami, T, Hiroce, V & Tucci, A (2007) Patterns of alcohol use between genders: a cross-cultural evaluation. *Journal of Affective Disorders* 102 (1) 265–275.

Kirksey, O, Harper, K, Thompson, S & Pringle, M (2004) Assessment of selected patient education materials of various chain pharmacies. *Journal of Health Communication* 9 (2) 91–93.

Kok, G, Schaalma, H, Ruiter, R A C & Empelen, P (2004) Intervention mapping: a protocol for applying health psychology theory to prevention programmes. *Journal of Health Psychology* 9 (1) 85–98.

Kools, M, van de Wiel, M W J, Ruiter, R A C, Crüts, A & Kok, G (2006) The effect of graphic organizers on subjective and objective comprehension of a health education text. *Health Education and Behaviour* 33 (6) 760–772.

Kornblau, I, Pearson, H & Breitkopf, C (2007) Demographic, behavioral, and physical correlates of body esteem among low-income female adolescents. *Journal of Adolescent Health* 41 (6) 566–570.

Kortesluoma, R L, Punamäki, R L & Nikkonen, M (2008) Hospitalized children drawing their pain: the contents and cognitive and emotional characteristics of pain drawings. *Journal of Child Health Care* 12 (4) 284–300.

Kraak, V & Pelletier, D L (1998) How marketers reach young consumers: implications for nutrition education and health promotion campaigns. *Family Economics and Nutrition Review* 11 (4) 31–41.

Kreps, G L & Maibach, E W (2009) Transdisciplinary science: the nexus between communication and public health. *Journal of Communication* 58 (3) 732–748.

Kreps, G L & Sparks, L (2008) Meeting the health literacy needs of immigrant populations. *Patient Education and Counseling* 71 (3) 328–332.

Kreuter, M W, Lukwago, S N, Bucholtz, D C, Clark, E M & Sanders-Thompson, V (2003) Achieving cultural appropriateness in health promotion programs: targeted and tailored approaches. *Health Education and Behaviour* 30 (2) 133–146.

Kulukulualani, M, Braun, K L & Tsark, J U (2008) Using a participatory 4 step protocol to develop culturally targeted cancer education brochures. *Health Promotion Practice* 9 (4) 344–355.

Kwok, C & Sullivan, G (2007) Heath seeking behaviours among Chinese-Australian women: implications for health promotion programmes. *Health* 11 (3) 401–415.

Larkey, L K & Gonzalez, J (2007) Storytelling for promoting colorectal cancer prevention and early detection among Latinos. *Patient Education and Counseling* 67 (3) 272–278.

Larson, EL, Wong-McLoughlin, J, & Ferng, Y (2009) Preferences among immigrant Hispanic women for written educational materials regarding upper respiratory infections. *Journal of Community Health* 34 (3) 202–209.

Lee, H (2007) Why sexual health promotion misses its audience. *Journal of Health Organization and Management* 21 (2) 205–219.

Levy, A S, Hawkes, A P & Rossie, G U (2007) Helmets for skiers and snowboarders: an injury prevention program. *Health Promotion Practice* 8 (3) 257–265.

Levy, S R, Anderson, E E, Issel, L M, Willis, M A, Dancy, B L, Jacobson, K M, et al. (2008) Using multilevel, multisource needs assessment data for planning community interventions. *Health Promotion Practice* 5 (1) 59–68.

Li, L, Rotheram-Borus, J, Lu, Y, Wu, Z, Lin, C & Guan, J (2009) Mass media and HIV/AIDS in China. *Journal of Health Communication* 14 (5) 424–438.

Lillie, T, Pulerwitz, J & Curbow, B (2009) Kenyan in-school youths' level of understanding of abstinence, being faithful, and consistent condom use terms: implications for HIV-prevention programs. *Journal of Health Communication* 14 (3) 276–292.

Lindsay, A C, Sussner, K N, Greaney, M L & Peterson, K E (2009) Influence of social context on eating, physical activity, and sedentary behaviors of Latina mothers and their preschool-age children. *Health Education & Behavior* 36 (1) 81–96.

Livingston, M & Room, R (2009) Variations by age and sex in alcohol-related problematic behaviour per drinking volume and heavier drinker occasion. *Drug and Alcohol Dependence* 101 (3) 169–175.

Lombardo, A P & Leger, Y A (2007) Thinking about 'Think Again' in Canada: assessing a social marketing HIV/AIDS prevention campaign. *Journal of Health Communication* 12 (4) 377–397.

Lovell. S, Kearns, R & A, Friesen, W (2007) Sociocultural barriers to cervical screening in South Auckland, New Zealand. *Social Science and Medicine* 65 (1) 138–150.

Lowther, M, Mutrie, N & Scott, E M (2007) Identifying key processes of exercise behaviour change associated with movement through the stages of exercise behaviour change. *Journal of Health Psychology* 12 (2) 261–272.

Lucas, K & Lloyd, B (2005) *Heath promotion: evidence and experience*. Sage, London.

Lyles, C M, Kay, L S, Crepaz, N, Herbst, J H, Passin, W F, Kim A S et al. (2007) Best evidence interventions: findings from a systematic review of HIV behavioural interventions for US populations at high risk 2000–2004. *American Journal of Public Health* 97 (1) 133–143.

Lynch, B M & Dunn, J (2003) Scoreboard advertising at sporting events as a health promotion medium. *Health Education Research* 18 (4) 488–492.

Ma, S, Hoang, M, Samet, J M, Wang, J, Mei, C, Xu, X et al. (2008) Myths and attitudes that sustain smoking in China. *Journal of Health Communication* 13 (7) 654–666.

Maddock, J, Silbanuz, A & Reger-Nash, B (2008) Formative research to develop a mass media campaign to increase physical activity and nutrition in a multiethnic state. *Journal of Health Communication* 13 (3) 208–218.

Manlove, J S, Terry-Humen, E, Ikramullah, E N, & Moore, K A (2006) The role of parent religiosity in teens' transitions to sex and contraception. *Journal of Adolescent Health* 39 (4) 578–587.

Mann, T, Sherman, D & Updegraff, J (2004) Dispositional motivations and message framing: a test of the congruency hypothesis in college students. *Health Psychology* 23 (3) 330–334.

Mao, Z & Wu, B (2007) Urban-rural age and gender differences in health behaviours in the Chinese population: findings from a survey in Hubei, China. *Public Health* 121 (10) 761–764.

Marcus, B H, Nigg, C R, Riebe, D & Forsyth, L H (2000) Interactive communication strategies: implications for population based physical activity promotion. *American Journal of Preventive Medicine* 19 (2) 121–126.

Marie Stopes (2009a) *Wilbert*, available at www.mariestopes.org.uk/documents/Mates.pdf and www.mariestopes.org.uk/documents/Clubbing.pdf

Marie Stopes (2009b) *Back Pocket Travel Guide*, available at www.mariestopes.org/documents/travelguide.pdf

Marlow, L A V, Waller, J, Evans, R E C & Wardle, J (2009) Predictors of interest in HPC vaccination: a study of British adolescents. *Vaccine* 27 (18) 2483–2488.

Maslen, A (2007) *Write to sell: the ultimate guide to great copywriting*. Marshall Cavendish Limited/Cyan Communications Ltd London.

Mason, T E & White, K M (2008) Applying an extended model of the theory of planned behaviour to breast self-examination. *Journal of Health Psychology* 13 (7) 946–955.

Mavalankar D & Abreu E (2002) Concepts and techniques for planning and implementing a program for renovation of an emergency obstetric care facility. *International Journal of Gynecology and Obstetrics* 78 (3) 263–273.

Mazor, K M & Billings-Gagliardi, S (2003) Does reading about stroke increase stroke knowledge? The impact of different print materials. *Patient Education and Counseling* 51 (3) 207–215.

Mbizvo, E (2006) Theatre – a force for health promotion. *The Lancet* 368 (S1) S30–31.

McEachan, R R C, Lawton, R J, Jackson, C, Conner, M & Lunt, J (2008) Evidence, theory and context: using intervention mapping to develop a worksite physical activity intervention. *BMC Public Health* 8 326 available at www.biomedcentral.com/1471-2458/8/326

McGilligan, C, McClenahan, C & Adamson, G (2009) Attitudes and intentions to performing testicular self-examination: utilizing an extended theory of planned behavior. *Journal of Adolescent Health* 44 (4) 404–406.

McKenna, K & Scott, J (2007) Do written education materials that use content and design principles improve older people's knowledge? *Australian Occupational Therapy Journal* 54 (2) 103–112.

McKenzie, J F, Neiger, B L & Smeltzer, J L (2005) *Planning, implementing and evaluating health promotion programmes: a primer*. Pearson, San Francisco.

McLaughlin, H G (1969) SMOG grading: a new readability formula. *Journal of Reading*, May, 639–646, available at, www.harrymclaughlin.com/SMOG_Readability_Formula_G._Harry_McLaughlin_(1969).pdf

McLaughlin, H G (2008) SMOG, available at www.harrymclaughlin.com/SMOG.htm

Meador, M G & Linnan, L A (2006) Using the PRECEDE model to plan men's health programs in a managed care setting. *Health Promotion Practice* 7 (2) 186–196.

Metropolitan Police (2008) *Which issues should your SNT tackle? You decide*, available at www.met.police.uk/campaigns/you_decide/you_decide.htm

Minc, A, Butler, T. & Gahan, G (2007) The jailbreak health project-incorporating a unique health programme for prisoners. *The International Journal of Drug Policy* 18 (5) 444–446.

Mitchell, K & Branigan, P (2000) Using focus groups to evaluate health promotion interventions. *Health Education* 100 (6) 261–268.

Mo, P K H & Mak, W W S (2008) Application of PRECEDE Model to understanding mental health promoting behaviours in Hong Kong. *Health Education and Behaviour* 35 (4) 574–587.

Moore, L V, Diez Roux, A V, Evenson, K, McGinn, A & Brines, S (2008) Availability of recreational resources in minority and low socioeconomic status areas. *American Journal of Preventive Medicine* 34 (1) 16–22.

Moss, H B, Kirby, S D & Donodeo, F (2009) Characterizing and reaching high risk drinkers using audience segmentation. *Alcoholism: Clinical and Experimental Research* 33 (1) 1336–1345.

Muthusamy, N, Levine, T R & Weber, R (2009) Scaring the already scared: some problems with HIV/AIDS fear appeals in Namibia. *Journal of Communication* 59 (2) 317–344.

Myhre, S L & Flora, J A (2000) HIV/AIDS communication campaigns: progress and prospects. *Journal of Health Communication* 5 (Suppl.) 29–45.

Närhi, U & Helakorpi, S (2007) Sources of medicine information in Finland. *Health Policy* 84 (1) 51–57.

National Cancer Institute (2003) *Clear and simple: developing effective print materials for low-literate readers*, available at www.nci.nih.gov/aboutnci/oc/clear-and-simple/allpages/print

National Institutes for Health (2008) *How to write easy-to-read health materials*, available at www.nlm.nih.gov/medlineplus/etr.html

National Literacy Trust (2009) *Readability – testing how easy a text is to read*, available from www.literacytrust.org.uk/campaign/SMOG.html

National Readership Survey (NRS) (2009) *National readership figures, Jan 08–Jun 09*, available at www.nrs.co.uk

National Social Marketing Council (NSMC) (2006a) *It's our health*, NSMC, London, available at www.nsmcentre.org.uk/

National Social Marketing Council (NSMC) (2006b) *Using social marketing as specified planned process. The 'total process planning model'*. NSMC, London available at www.nsmcentre.org.uk/

NIACE (2009) *Readability SMOG calculation*, available at www.niace.org.uk/development-research/readability

NICE (2007) *Behaviour change: the most appropriate means of genetic and specific interventions to support attitude and behaviour change at individual and population levels*, available at: http://guidance.nice.org.uk/PH6

NICE (2008) *Mental well being of older people*, available at: http://guidance.nice.org.uk/PH16

Noar, S M, Palmgreen, P, Chabot, M, Dobransky, N & Zimmerman, R S (2009) A ten year systematic review of HIV/AIDS mass communication campaigns: have we made progress? *Journal of Health Communication* 14 (1) 15–42.

Nonnemaker, J M, McNeely, C A & Blum, R W (2003) Public and private domains of religiosity and adolescent health risk behaviors: evidence from the National Longitudinal Study of Adolescent Health. *Social Science and Medicine* 57 (11) 2049–2054.

Nonoyama, M, Tsurugi, Y, Shirai, C, Ishikawa, Y & Horiguchi, M (2007) Influences of sex related information for STD prevention. *Journal of Adolescent Health* 36 (5) 442–445.

Nutbeam, D (2008) The evolving concept of health literacy. *Social Science and Medicine* 67 (12) 2072–2078.

Nutbeam, D & Harris, E (2004) *Theory in a nutshell: A guide to health promotion theory, 2nd edition*. McGraw-Hill, London.

Oetzel, J (2007) Hispanic women's preferences for breast health information: subjective cultural influences on source, message, and channel. *Health Communication* 21 (3) 223–233.

ONS (2004) *Smoking & drinking – Bangladeshi men have highest smoking rates*. Office for National Statistics, London, available at www.statistics.gov.uk_

ONS (2008) *General Household Survey: Smoking and drinking among adults 2007*. Office for National Statistics, London, available at www.statistics.gov.uk

Otero-Sabogal, R, Stewart, S, Shema, S J & Pasick, R J (2007) Ethnic differences in decisional balance and stages of mammography adoption. *Health Education & Behavior* 34 (2) 278–296.

Paek, H, Lee, B, Salmon, C & T, Witte, K (2008) The contextual effects of gender norms, communication and social capital on family planning behaviours in Uganda: a multilevel approach. *Health Education Behaviour* 35 (4) 461–477.

Parker, R M, & Gazmararian, J A (2003) Health literacy: essential for health communication. *Journal of Health Communication* 8 (Suppl 1) 116–118.

Patten, C A, Decker, P A, Dornelas, E A, Barbagallo, J, Rock, E, Offord, K P et al. (2008) Changes in readiness to quit and self-efficacy among adolescents receiving a brief office intervention for smoking cessation. *Psychology, Health and Medicine* 13 (3) 326–336.

Pearce, A, Kirk, C, Cummins, S, Collins, M, Elliman, D, Connolly, A M et al. (2009) Gaining children's perspectives: a multiple method approach to explore environmental influences on healthy eating and physical activity. *Health & Place* 15 (2) 614–621.

Peattie, S (2007) The internet as a medium for communicating with teenagers. *Social Marketing Quarterly* XIII (2) 21–46.

Peddecord, K M, Jacobson, I G, Engelberg, M, Kwizera, L, Macias, V & Gustafson, K W (2008) Can movie theatre advertisements promote health behaviours? Evaluation of a flu vaccination pilot campaign. *Journal of Health Communication* 13 (6) 596–613.

Pepall, E, Earnest, J & James, R (2006) Understanding community perceptions of health and social needs in a rural Balinese village: results of a rapid appraisal. *Health Promotion International* 22 (1) 44–52.

Peters, G Y, Kok, G & Abraham, C (2007) Social cognitive determinants of ecstasy use to target in evidence-based interventions: a meta-analytical review. *Addiction* 103 (1) 109–118.

Petti, S & Scully, C (2007) Oral cancer knowledge and awareness: primary and secondary effects of an information leaflet. *Oral Oncology* 43 (4) 408–415.

Philpott, A, Knerr, W & Boydell, V (2006) Pleasure and prevention: when good sex is safer sex. *Reproductive Health Matters* 14 (28) 23–31.

Piko, B F & Bak, J (2006) Children's perceptions of health and illness; images and lay concepts in preadolescence. *Health Education Research* 21 (5) 643–653.

Pinfold, J V (1999) Analysis of different communication channels for promoting hygiene behaviour. *Health Education Research* 14 (5) 629–639.

Pluhar, E I, DiLorio, C K & McCarthy, F (2008) Correlates of sexuality communication among mothers and 6–12 year old children. *Child Care Health and Development* 34 (3) 283–290.

Porto, M P (2007) Fighting AIDS among adolescent women: effects of a public communication campaign in Brazil. *Journal of Health Communication* 12 (2) 121–132.

Potvin, L, Cargo, M, McComber, A M, Delormier, T & Macaulay, A C (2003) Implementing participatory intervention and research in communities: lessons from the Kahnawake schools diabetes prevention project in Canada. *Social Science and Medicine* 56 (6) 1295–1305.

Povlsen, L, Olsen, B & Ladelund, S (2005) Educating families from ethnic minorities in type 1 diabetes – experiences from a Danish intervention study. *Patient Education and Counseling* 59 (2) 164–170.

Prochaska, J O & Diclemente, C C (1983) Stages and processes of self-change in smoking: toward an integrative model of change. *Journal of Consulting and Clinical Psychology* 51 (3) 390–395.

Prochaska, J O & Velicer W F (1997) The transtheoretical model of health behavior change. *American Journal of Health Promotion* 12 (1) 38–48.

QUIT (2007) *Don't overdo it* poster, available at www.quit.org.uk/

Raine, T, Minnis, A M & Padian, N S (2003) Determinants of contraceptive method among young women at risk for unintended pregnancy and sexually transmitted infections. *Contraception* 68 (1) 19–25.

Rajar (2009) *Radio listening figures*, available at www.rajar.co.uk

Ramey, S L, Downing, N R & Knoblauch, A (2008) Developing strategic interventions to reduce cardiovascular disease risk among law enforcement officers. *American Association of Occupational Health* 56 (2) 54–62.

Redfern, J, Rudd, A D, Charles, D A & Wolfe, C M (2008) Stop stroke: development of an innovative intervention to improve risk factor management after stroke. *Patient Education and Counseling* 72 (2) 201–209.

Reger, B, Cooper, L, Booth-Butterfield, P, Smith, H, Bauman, A, Wootan, M. et al. (2002) Wheeling walks: a community campaign using paid media to encourage walking among sedentary older adults. *Preventive Medicine* 35 (3) 285–292.

Reinaerts, E, De Nooijer, J & De Vries, N K (2008) Using intervention mapping for system-atic development of two school-based interventions aimed at increasing children's fruit and vegetable intake. *Health Education* 108 (4) 301–320.

Reinert, B, Carver, V, Range, L M & Pike, C (2008) Collecting health data with youth at faith-based institutions: lessons learned. *Health Promotion Practice* 9 (1) 8–75.

Rios-Ellis, B, Frates, J, D'Anna, L H, Dwyer, M, Lopez-Zetina, J & Ugarte, C (2008) Addressing the need for access to culturally and linguistically appropriate HIV/AIDS prevention for Latinos. *Journal of Immigrant and Minority Health* 10 (5) 445–460.

Ritchie, D, Schulz, S & Bryce, A (2007) One size fits all? A process evaluation – the turn of the story in smoking cessation. *Public Health* 121 (5) 341–347.

Roe, K & Roe, K (2004) Dialogue boxes: a tool for collaborative process evaluation. *Health Promotion Practice* 5 (2) 138–150.

Rose, T A, Worrall, L E & McKenna, K T (2003) The effectiveness of aphasia-friendly principles for printed health education materials for people with aphasia following stroke. *Aphasiology* 17 (10) 947–963.

Rothman, A J (2004) 'Is there nothing so practical than a good theory?' Why innovations and advances in health behaviour change will arise if interventions are used to test and refine theory. *International Journal of Behavioural Nutrition and Physical Activity*, 1:11, available at www.ijbnpa.org/content/1/1/11

Rothman, A J, Martino, S C, Bedell, B T, Detweiler, J T & Salovey, P (1999) The systematic influence of gain and loss framed messages on interest in and use of different types of health behaviour. *Personality and Social Psychology Bulletin* 25 (11) 1355–1369.

Ruel, M T, Menon, P, Habicht, J, Loechl, C, Bergeron, G, Pelto, G et al. (2008) Age based preventive targeting of food assistance and behaviour change and communication for reduction of childhood under nutrition in Haiti: a cluster randomised trial. *The Lancet*, 371, Feb 16, 588–595.

Russell, M L, Thurston, W E & Henderson, E A (2003) Theory and models for planning and evaluating institutional influenza prevention and control programs. *American Journal of Infection Control* 31 (6) 336–341.

Saks, M & Allsop, J (2008) *Researching health*. Sage, London.

Samaritans (2008) *Media guidelines for reporting suicide and self-harm*, available at www.samaritans.org

Saunders, R P, Evans, M H & Joshi, P (2005) Developing a process evaluation place for assessing health promotion program implementation: a how to guide. *Health Promotion Practice* 6 (2) 134–147.

Sawney, F (2006) Theatre in health promotion 86–96, in Macdowall, W, Bonell, C & Davis, M (2007) *Health promotion practice*. Open University Press, Maidenhead.

Schouten, B C, Van den Putte, B, Pasmans, M & Meeuwesen, L (2007) Parent-adolescent communication about sexuality: the role of adolescent beliefs, subject norm and perceived behavioural control. *Patient Education and Counseling* 66 (1) 75–83.

Scratchmedia (2009) *Readability – making web pages easy to read*, available at www.webdesignfromscratch.com/basics/readability.php

Shahid, S, Finn, L, Bessarab, D & Thompson, S C (2009) Understanding, beliefs and perspectives of aboriginal people in Western Australia about cancer and its impact on access to cancer services. *BMC Health Services Research*, 9 132, available at www.biomedcentralcom/1472–6963/9/132

Shuval, K, Weissblueth, E, Brezis, M, Araida, A, Faridi, Z, Ali, A et al. (2008) The role of culture, environment and religion in the promotion of physical activity among Arab Israelis. *Preventing Chronic Disease* 5 (3), available at www.cdc.gov/dcd/issues/2008/jul/07_0104.htm

Siminoff, L A, Graham, G C & Gordon, N H (2006) Cancer communication patterns and the influence of patient characteristics: disparities in information-giving and affective behaviours. *Patient Education and Counseling* 62 (3) 255–360.

Sivaram, S, Johnson, S, Bentley, M E, Srikrishnan, A K, Latkin, C A, Go, V F et al. (2007) Exploring 'wine shops' as a venue for HIV prevention interventions in urban India. *Journal of Urban Health* 84 (4) 563–576.

Sohl, S J & Moyer, A (2007) Tailored interventions to promote mammography screening: a meta-analytic review. *Preventive Medicine* 45 (4) 252–261.

Solberg, L I, Maciosek, M V & Edwards, N M (2008) Primary care intervention to reduce alcohol misuse. *American Journal of Preventive Medicine* 34 (2) 143–152.

Soto Mas, F G, Kane, W M, Going, S, Ford, E S, Marshall, J R, Staten, L K et al. (2000) Camine Con Nosotros: connecting theory and practice for promoting physical activity among Hispanic women. *Health Promotion Practice* 1 (2) 178–187.

Soul City Institute (2009) *Soul city*, available at www.soulcity.org.za/

SPINZ (Suicide Prevention in New Zealand) (2009) *SPINZ*, available at www.twitter.com/suicidenz.

Springston, J K & Champion, V L (2004) Public relations and cultural aesthetics: designing health brochures. *Public Relations Review* 30 (4) 483–491.

Starkey, F & Orme, J (2001) Evaluation of a primary school drug drama project: methodological issues and key findings. *Health Education Research* 16 (5) 609–622.

Sturcke, J (2009) Cancer tests go up after Goody diagnosis *The Guardian*, Tues 17 Dec., available at www.guardian.co.uk/media/2009/feb/17/cancer-tests-jade-goody

Suggs, L S (2006) A 10 year retrospective of research in new technologies for health communication. *Journal of Health Communication* 11 (1) 61–74.

Suggs, L S & McIntyre, C (2009) Are we there yet? An examination of online tailored health communication. *Health Education and Behaviour* 36 (2) 278–288.

Sun, A, Zhang, J, Tsoh, J, Wong-Kim, E & Chow, E (2007) The effectiveness in utilizing Chinese media to promote breast health among Chinese women. *Journal of Health Communication* 12 (2) 157–171.

SURL (2002) *A comparison of online fonts which size and type is best*, Wichita State University, US available at http://psychology.wichita.edu/surl/usabilitynews/41/online-text.htm

Swaim, R A, Barner, J C & Brown, C M (2008) The relationship of calcium intake and exercise to osteoporosis health beliefs in postmenopausal women. *Research in Social and Administrative Pharmacy* 4 (2) 153–163.

Synder, L B (2001) How effective are mediated health campaigns? 181–192, in Rice, R E & Atkin, C K (eds) *Public communication campaigns, 3rd edition*. Sage, London.

TalktoFrank (2009a) *Frankbot*, available at http://talktofrank.com/

TalktoFrank (2009b) *Cannabis*, available at http://talktofrank.com/cannabis.aspx

Tanaka, Y, Kunii, O, Hatano, T & Wakai, S (2008) Knowledge, attitude and practice (KAP) of HIV prevention and HIV infection risks among Congolese refugees in Tanzania. *Health and Place* 14 (3) 434–452.

Tanvatanakul, V, Amado, J & Saowakontha, S (2007) Management of communication channels for health information in the community. *Health Education Journal* 66 (2) 173–178.

Terblanche-Smit, M & Terblanche, N S (2009) Race and attitude formation in HIV/Aids fear advertising. *Journal of Business Research* (In press).

Thackery, R & Neiger, B L (2009) A multidirectional communication model: implications for social marketing practice. *Health Promotion Practice* 10 (2) 171–175.

Thackery, R, Neiger, B & Hanson, C L (2007) Developing a promotional strategy: important questions for social marketing. *Health Promotion Practice* 8 (4) 332–336.

The Communications Network (2008) *Are we there yet?* Available at www.comnetwork.org

The Office of Minority Health (2007) *HHS fact-sheet: minority health disparities at a glance*, available at http://www.omhrc.gov/templates/content.aspx?ID=2139

The Prostate Cancer Charity (2009) *Movember*, available at www.movember.com

Thesite.org (2009) *Sexual myths*, available at www.thesite.org/sexandrelationships/sexuality/awareness/sexmyths.

Thinkbox (2009) *BHF: watch your own heart attack* available at www.thinkbox.tv/server/show/concasestudy.1395

Thomas, M, Gillespie, W, Krauss, J, Harrison, S, Medeiros, R, Hawkins, M et al. (2005) Focus group data as a tool in assessing effectiveness of a hand hygiene campaign. *American Journal of Infection Control* 33 (6) 368–373.

Tian, Y & Robinson, J D (2008) Incidental health information use and media complementarity: a comparison of senior and non senior cancer patients. *Patient Education and Counseling* 71 (3) 340–344.

Tilson, E C, Sanchez, V, Ford, C L, Smurzynski, M, Leone, P A, Fox, K K et al. (2004) Barriers to asymptomatic screening and other STD services for adolescents and young adults: focus group discussions. *BMC Public Health*, 4:21, available at www.biomed-central.com/1471-2458/4/21

Time to change (2009) *Time to change*, available at www.time-to-change.org.uk/home/

Tones, K & Green J (2004) *Health promotion: planning and strategy.* Sage, London.

Tortolero, S R, Markham, C M, Parcel, G S, Peters, R J, Escobar-Chaves, S L, Basen-Engquist, K et al. (2005) Using intervention mapping to adapt an effective HIV, sexually transmitted disease and pregnancy prevention program for high risk minority youth. *Health Promotion Practice* 6 (3) 286–298.

Trident (2009a) *Stop the guns*, available at www.stoptheguns.org/

Trident (2009b) *Drop the weapons*, available at www.droptheweapons.org/

Tufano, J T & Karras, B T (2005) Mobile ehealth interventions for obesity: a timely opportunity to leverage convergence trends. *Journal of Medical Internet Research*, 7 (5) e58, available at www.jmir.org/2005/4/e1/

UNESCO (2001) Charting the progress of populations – adult literacy, available at www.un.org/esa/population/publications/charting/11.pdf

Utzinger, J, Wyss, K, Moto, D D, Tanner, M & Singer, B H (2004) Community health outreach program of the Chad-Cameroon Petroleum Development and Pipeline Project. *Clinical Occupational Environmental Medicine* 4 (1) 9–26.

Uutela, A, Absetz, P, Nissinen, A, Valve, R, Talja & M Fogleholm, M (2004) Health psychological theory in promoting population health in Päijät-Häme, Finland: first steps toward a type 2 diabetes prevention study. *Journal of Health Psychology* 9, (1) 73–84.

Valente, T W (2001) Evaluating communication campaigns, 105–124, in Rice, R E & Atkin, C K (eds) *Public communication campaigns, 3rd edition*. Sage, London.

Vallance, J K, Courneya, K S, Taylor, L M, Plotnikoff, R C & Mackey, J R (2008) Development and evaluation of a theory-based physical activity guidebook for breast cancer survivors. *Health Education and Behaviour* 35 (2) 174–189.

Vallance, J K, Taylor, L M & Lavallee, C (2008) Suitability and readability assessment of educational print resources related to physical activity: implications and recommendations for practice. *Patient Education and Counseling* 72 (2) 342–349.

Vallely, A, Shagi, C, Kasindi, S, Desmond, N, Lees, S & Chiduo, B (2007) The benefits of participatory methodology to develop effective community dialogue in the context of a microbicide trial feasibility study in Mwanza, Tanzania. *BMC Public Health*. Jul. 7 (147) 133, available at www.biomedcentral.com/1471-2458/7/133

Victor, R G, Ravenell, J E, Freeman, A, Bhat, D G, Storm, J S, Shafiq, M et al. (2009) A barber-based intervention for hypertension in African American men: design of a randomised control trial. *American Heart Journal* 157 (1) 30–36.

Wang, B, Li, X, McGuire, J, Kamali, V, Fang, X & Stanton, B (2009) Understanding the dynamics of condom use among female sex workers in China. *Sexually Transmitted Diseases* 36 (3) 134–140.

Wang, S, Moss, J R & Hiller, J E (2005) Applicability and transferability of interventions in evidence-based public health. *Health Promotion International* 21 (1) 76–83.

Wasilewski, R M, Mateo, P & Sidorovsky, P (2008) Preventing work related musculoskeletal disorders within supermarket cashiers: an ergonomic training program based on the theoretical framework of the PRECEDE-PROCEED model. *Work* 28 (1) 23–31.

Waters, R D, Burnett, E, Lamm, A & Lucas, J (2009) Engaging stakeholders through social networking: how non profit organizations are using Facebook. *Public Relations Review* 35 (2) 102–106.

Weintraub, D, Maliski, S L, Fink, A, Choe, S & Litwin, M S (2004) Suitability of prostate cancer education materials: applying a standardized assement tool to current available materials. *Patient Education and Counseling* 55 (2) 275–280.

Wellings, K & Macdowall, W (2006) Evaluating mass media approaches, 145–166, in Thorogood, M & Coombes, Y (eds) *Evaluating health promotion*, Oxford University Press, Oxford.

Westaway, M S & Viljkoen, E (2000) Health and hygiene knowledge, attitudes and behaviour. *Health and Place* 6 (1) 25–32.

White, A & Cash, K (2004) The state of men's health in Western Europe. *Journal of Men's Health* 1 (1) 60–66.

White, K M, Robinson, N G, Young, R M, Anderson, P J, Hyde, M K, Greenbank, S, et al. (2008) Testing an extended theory of planned behaviour to predict young people's sun safety in a high risk area. *British Journal of Health Psychology* 13 (3) 435–448.

Whitelaw, S, Baxendale, A, Bryce, C, Machardy, L, Young, I & Witney, E (2001) 'Settings' based health promotion: a review. *Health Promotion International* 16 (4) 339–353.

Whittingham, J R D, Ruiter, R A C, Castermans, D, Huberts, A & Kok, G (2008) Designing effective health education materials: experimental pre-testing of a theory based brochure to increase knowledge. *Health Education Research* 23 (3) 414–426.

Whysall, Z J, Haslam, C & Haslam, R A (2007) Developing the Stage of Change approach for the reduction of work-related musculoskeletal disorders. *Journal of Health Psychology* 12 (1) 184–197.

Wiedemann, A U, Lippke, S, Reuter, R, Schüz, B, Ziegelmann, J P & Schwarzer, R (2009) Prediction of stage transitions in fruit and vegetable intake. *Health Education Research* 24 (4) 596–607.

Wiehagen, T, Caito, N M, Saunders Thompson, V, Casey, C M, Weaver, N L, Jupka, K & Kreuter, M W (2007) Applying projective techniques to formative research in health community development. *Health Promotion Practice* 8 (2) 164–172.

Wiggins, M, Bonell, C & Burchett, H (2007) Evaluating health promotion, 207–219, in MacDowall, W, Bonell, C & Davis, M (2007) *Health promotion practice*. Open University Press, Maidenhead.

Wilkin, H A & Ball-Rokeach, S J (2006) Reaching at risk groups: the importance of health story telling in Los Angeles Latino media. *Journalism* 7 (3) 299–320.

Willging, C E, Helitzer, D & Thompson, J (2006) 'Sharing wisdom': lessons learned during the development of a diabetes prevention intervention for urban American Indian women. *Evaluation and Program Planning* 29 1130–1140.

Witte, K & Allen, M (2000) A meta-analysis of fear appeals: implications for effective public health campaigns. *Health Education & Behavior* 27 (5) 591–615.

Wolfers, M E G, Hoek, C, Brug, J & Zwart, O (2007) Using intervention mapping to develop a programme to prevent sexual transmitted infections, including HIV, among heterosexual migrant men. *BMC Health* 7 (141), available at http://www.biomedcentral.com/1471-2458/7/141

Wong, L P (2009) HPV information needs, educational messages and channel of delivery preferences: views from developing country with multiethnic populations. *Vaccine* 27 (9) 1410–1415.

Woodrow, C, Watson, E, Rozmovits, L, Parker, R & Austoker, J (2007) Public perceptions of communicating information about bowel cancer screening. *Health Expectations* 11 (1) 16–25.

WRAP (2006) *Improving the performance of waste diversion schemes: A good practice guide to monitoring and evaluation*, available at www.wrap.org.uk

Wright, A, McGorry, P D, Harris, M G, Jorm, A F & Pennell, K (2006) Development and evaluation of a youth mental health community awareness campaign: the compass strategy. *BMC Public Health*, 6: 215, available at http://www.biomedcentral.com/1471-2458/6/215

Wynn, L L, Foster, A M & Trussell, J (2009) Can I get pregnant from oral sex? Sexual health misconceptions in emails to a reproductive health website. *Contraception* 79 (2) 91–7.

Yancey, A K, McCarthy, W J, Taylor, W C, Merlo, A, Gewa, C, Weber, M D et al. (2004) The Los Angeles Lift Off: a social cultural environmental change intervention to integrate physical activity into the workplace. *Preventive Medicine* 38 (6) 848–856.

Yeo, M, Berzins, S, Addington, D (2007) Development of an early psychosis public education program using the PRECEDE-PROCEED model. *Health Education Research* 22 (5) 639–647.

Author's note

Internet references were correct at the last date checked: September 2009. If a website link no longer exists you are advised to locate the original site (i.e. WHO, Department of Health, etc.) and search for the document from the original location.

Index

NOTE: page numbers in *italic type* refer to figures and tables.